# DESPERATELY SEEKING SEMEN
## *My Rogue Route to Solo Motherhood*

HAYLEY HENDRIX

HAYLEY HENDRIX

Hayley Hendrix
Brisbane, Australia,
www.kbuti.com

Cover design by Amygdala Design
ISBN: 978-0-6484950-0-0

*To all women who are desperately seeking semen*

# CONTENTS

Foreword ................................................................................ vii

Acknowledgements ............................................................... ix

Prologue .............................................................................. xi

## *PART I*

Chapter 1 Flying to Meet Mr. Stork ................................... 2

Chapter 2 A Decade of Me Instead of We (AKA My Thirties) ...... 6

Chapter 3 SHIPS - The Life Changing Three ........................ 14

Chapter 4 The Life Crash.................................................... 30

## *PART II*

Chapter 5 The Back Story .................................................. 35

Chapter 6 Nature or Nurture ............................................. 39

Chapter 7 Pull the Ex Ripcord .......................................... 45

Chapter 8 Sista's Without Misters ...................................... 50

Chapter 9 Seed Dating ....................................................... 56

Chapter 10 Donor Swimmers over Tinder Dinners.................. 61

Chapter 11 Girl Gone Rogue .............................................. 76

Chapter 12 Gone Fishin'..................................................... 92

Chapter 13 Mr. Stork.......................................................... 104

Chapter 14 Y? .................................................................... 112

## *PART III*

Chapter 15 Needles and Haystacks ..................................... 121

Chapter 16 CONtroversy .................................................... 127

Chapter 17 The Deed.......................................................... 131

Chapter 18 Time Bending Tips ........................................... 137

Chapter 19 My BFP ;).......................................................... 144

# PART IV

Chapter 20 Child Free in the City ............................... 151
Chapter 21 Man of The House ..................................... 174
Chapter 22 In the Present with My Present ................ 180
Chapter 23 Genetic Connections ................................. 185
Chapter 24 The Donor Daily ....................................... 191
Chapter 25 Looking Back ............................................ 198
Epilogue Looking Ahead ............................................ 202

Glossary ...................................................................... 206
Find Out More ............................................................ 210
Suicide Crisis Support ................................................ 211
References ................................................................... 212

# Foreword

*HAYLEY IS A SPECIAL GIRL.* No challenge is too big for her. She wanted to have a healthy child. Superficially this should not present a problem as she is a very attractive, fit, and healthy young woman.

However, there was one major obstacle to achieving this goal: she needed healthy sperm from someone with good genetics. This book is about the innovative way she achieved that goal.

The task of producing a child is not as simple as it sounds even for a couple who believe they are perfectly healthy. Currently in Australia, about 30% of couples who want to have a child are unable to conceive a child naturally, and by 2030, the percentage is forecast to increase to 50%.

The major reason for this is one or both partners have the gene for food intolerance and their immune system has been hypersensitized by the food they eat, switching on autoimmune conditions such as PCOS and endometriosis in the female and creating Immunoglobulin G in the semen of the male that compromises the motility of the sperm.

Sadly, most people do not recognise they have food intolerance, and if they did know, they would not understand the link between food and infertility.

Thankfully there is a simple solution to overcoming the food intolerance that allows the autoimmune conditions to be switched off and activates repair to the reproductive system. Unfortunately, that does not make semen appear from heaven, but at least when good quality semen is found, and the female's reproductive system has been optimised, success will follow.

Hayley overcame her problem, and then set herself the task of helping other people with the same problem.

This wonderful book is a part of her program to help people throughout the world produce full-term babies even when one part of the equation is missing – healthy sperm.

Clifford Hawkins Sc Ph Sc

# Acknowledgements

*I AM FOREVER GRATEFUL TO* my friends who are my soul sisters, Cheryl and Kim, who not only supported me in every way on this wild ride but climbed aboard and held my hand. Their wanting of this for me was equal to my deep longing to become a mother. Thanks ladies for standing by my side during those baby scans, tolerating my nails gouging those same hands of yours in the birthing suite, and being part of this very personal, yet public roller coaster.

Sue and Frank, for giving me a nest so I could birth two babies this year. Carmen, for being there when it dawned on me that single motherhood was my reality. Your presence along this path has always been felt. Georgie, for showing me why I needed to keep on going. Professor Cliff Hawkins, for giving me the OK in every way.

Thank you Adam Hooper for normalising this path and creating one of the most accessible social donor hubs for women all across Australia.

A massive thank you to my interviewees, some of whose names and locations I've changed to protect their identities—John Lyndsay Mayger, The late John Cady, Jim Smith, Michael, Caitlin, Katrina, Laura, Christian, Juan, Matt C, Tracey and Annie for sharing your stories and wisdom with me to include here. Stephen Page for all his insight and expertise. All the SHIPS that sailed in and out of my life. Dr Hayes, the midwives and doctors at The Royal Women's Hospital in Brisbane, Pim for blessing us with his name, and most notably my Mum who was brave enough to share her story.

I am blessed to have so many wing-women scattered all over the globe who've reached out to me during my pregnancy offering their love and support. Thank you for your friendship and holding me in life even if we don't see each other in the flesh very often. You know who you are!

Rachelle, you are a gem shining bright on the other side of the planet. Without your editing prowess, this book would not exist in its current form. I owe you so much for opening me up to telling this story in a way I could not have fathomed a year ago.

And to my donor, for his generous gift for whom I'm forever grateful and making this such a pleasant and wonderful journey.

# Prologue

*"Women don't have to be defined by others. We have the power to define ourselves: by telling our own stories, in our own words, with our own voices." - Sarah Kay, poet*

*Mr Stork: When could you be here?*
*Hayley: A few hours*
*Mr Stork: Why not? Let's do it!*
*Hayley: Ok I'll need to see your hard copy ID mister ☺ I can arrive at 5 pm. Booking hotel now...prob Mantra hotel. Does that work for you?*

Some of us grew up dreaming about the house with the white picket fence, the two kids, the gorgeous partner standing by one's side. You know the one—that scene that is on a loop in your mind—the one that's not real. Well, for many of us it's not. I never dreamed of the white picket fence, but when I worked with a life coach back in 2005 this is what I visualised:

*'In five year's time, I will be: Watching my husband holding our 8-month-old baby in the hammock at our stunning modern boho home that overlooks the ocean as the sun sets. It was a warm, balmy afternoon and I pinched myself so I knew what I was seeing was real.'*

Boom! The wake-up thump. Twelve years later and none of that had happened thus far. It's what then happened over the following 18 months that has me tapping away on my keyboard to put this book together.

Did I ever see myself struggling to find someone to make a baby with? An emphatic NO. Did I ever see myself here? NO. Well, maybe not exactly like this. Actually, if I am completely honest with myself, deep down I was probably destined to roll solo as a mother at some point. It's in my DNA.

Still, I had absolutely no idea it would turn out quite as it has.

# PART I

*Chapter 1*
# Flying to Meet Mr. Stork

*"Life begins at the end of your comfort zone."*
*- Neale Donald Walsch, author*

THIS ISN'T JUST ANY VIRGIN flight; it's my maiden Virgin flight. I am a donee virgin. But in just a few hours, I will be knocked up. Or I am hoping to be by my internet sperm donor, who I refer to as Mr Stork.

Flying high at thirty thousand feet in the air, all I could think about was how I needed thirty thousand tails injected into me with just two feet in the air.

Kim and Chez, my two closest girlfriends and wing women who run my 'Desperately Seeking Semen (DSS) Crusade Committee', had just coordinated my hasty trip south. With military precision, all my meticulous research and planning had finally aligned, yet I was still hesitant to make that final jump. It was my discussions with them and their moral support that helped me finally take that last minute leap. Chez managed to secure me a seat on a flight, and Kim promptly bundled me into the car and drove me to the airport.

Shit got real. Real fast.

Now, I was on my way to Melbourne to meet Mr Stork in the flesh. A stark contrast, or should I say, a stork contrast, from my plane ride back to Australia after my most recent break up with Ian, my boyfriend of whom I was with during my fast depreciating final fertile years. I had finally split with him for good and had come completely undone.

We had just zoomed around Europe together in a week of 'taking care of business'. We flew so fast on four wheels from the UK through France, burned past Bern across Switzerland into Italy where we enjoyed the sights of Lake Como from our hotel window, after flying over the Alps in our rented Toyota Corolla. Venice was done in a day before we took off south for Monaco for one night, then headed back up through France via Lyon, before making our way back to the UK. I think we saw more of the insides of McDonald's during our service stops, which included email, phone and coffee refuelling as well as the dumping of any excess fluids.

Five days of crazy driving, being cooped up in a box on four wheels, with my cheeks riding in the back seat, my fingernails clenching the car seat, one eye taking in the scenery through the rear vision mirror while the other followed the moving dot on the map. Dizzy Siri, teamed with my spidey senses, did our best to navigate us through foreign cities with frustration, anger, confusion and sadness, all pointing fingers in all directions. Her prissy English voice couldn't even drown out the silent emotional discourse.

Back then, our satellite navigation was more scrambled than my own head trying to figure out where we were, but now there was nothing confusing about the flight from Brisbane to Melbourne. The hotel was booked. The shuttle arranged. Donor enroute. Decisive and ready, I was heading very clearly in the right direction.

Mr Stork and I had arranged to meet at a hotel close to Tullamarine Airport so I could catch an early flight back to Brisbane the following day. It was dark by the time the plane landed, and I caught the hotel shuttle, which was about to take off when I finally found the right stand to catch it from. Vacillating right up until an hour before the plane left, I didn't have any luggage with me—just an oversized handbag that had a few toiletries, a change of underwear, my pyjamas and a clean top for the morning, all thrown in. I couldn't help but feel a little like Alex Goran meeting up with Ryan Bingham to start one of many travel encounters in the 2009 movie "Up in the Air".

Alex wasn't in it for the baby, though. She already had that taken care of despite Ryan being blissfully unaware of that minor detail. I, on the other hand, was. And I was mentally and emotionally prepared to get on a plane every month to rendezvous with my Mr Stork if I had to. I was on a long-haul pregnancy mission to do as many cycles it would take for just one slippery little sucker to puncture one of my rapidly deflating fertile balloons.

Up until that point, I had dated pretty much every kind of guy out there—from TV network and media types to professional sportsmen to a spiritually enlightened being. I had even dated an accountant! Some rode motorbikes; others, highfalutin four-wheeled numbers. One guy actually road his beat-up, motor less road bike over to pick me up. Until then, I hadn't dinkied since I was fourteen. I haven't done so again. They were all now just stories from my past only brought back to life when my mind was able to resurrect and dust off a badly filed memory, and when my breath and vocal folds met.

As I travelled towards my destination at around 500 knots, and my belly in one giant knot, these memories had surfaced for some reason. Kind of like my mind was throwing out these events in frozen snippets and pixelated frames just like a computer does when the hard-drive decides to cark it because it had been so bogged down with stuff I didn't even know it was stored. Some were in a chokehold as they really didn't need any oxygen to come to life ever again.

It was like I was doing a quick clean to make room for my second life act, as Jane Fonda referred to it in her 2011 TEDx Talk 'Life's Third Act'. In her speech, she discussed how life is generally viewed as being an arch where we ascend until midlife (First act) and then after that, it's just a downhill ride (Second act).

She points out that we're living on average 30 years longer today than our great-grandparents which by comparison has added an entire second adult lifetime to our lifespan (Third act). So rather than just having an up and down or two acts, she views life as a staircase with these extra years as a chance to live these bonus decades to the fullest; perhaps even to make a 'life review'.

My first act 'up' was done. It could not be changed. It could, however, be reviewed and used later on in life to give clarity and new meaning. But I didn't have to wait for my third act to do what the Fabulous Ms Fonda was suggesting. As I edged closer to what potentially would be the biggest point of change, and start of my Second Act, these past actions and memories were able to tell me a little more about who I was now. How I got me here.

As I reflected on my Act One, I was so excited and nervous sitting in my seat looking out to the clouds. I had so much hope riding on this trip, yet no idea how it would all unfold.

# Chapter 2

# A Decade of Me Instead of We (AKA My Thirties)

*"You are only young once, and if you work it right, once is enough."*
*- Joe E. Lewis, performer*

IT WAS AUGUST OF 2015, and I had a one-way ticket to Albany, Australia. I was mortified that my expat life was over and I was on a plane heading back to my mum.

I had been living in the US since 2006 working in and out of TV production, feeding my entrepreneurial spirit with grandiose thoughts and a lifestyle vision that was so sweet any Michelin star chef would want to taste it.

A Perth girl, I'd been living in Sydney for ten years prior having moved there to study journalism and then work my way up from logging sports tapes at Channel 7 to a cushy little on-camera gig in Kids TV on a rival network. I relocated from Sydney to Brisbane for 12 months working on Network Ten's "Totally Wild" before relocating back down again 12 months later. Kids TV wasn't a normal job; it was a role where I got to do as I would say, "everything I never got to do as a teenager."

One day I would jump out of a plane, the next I would spend the morning abseiling down cliffs, then in the afternoon, I would be out on the harbour saving injured turtles. It was a sweet gig that took me from talking salty barrels with Australian surfing legends to getting skiing tips from up-and-coming Olympians while freezing to death on crisp snow-capped mountains.

Although it was a good path to lead me to bigger or other TV opportunities, I had itchy feet, a broken heart from Trey, a man I wanted to marry and was feeling uninspired in life and work. It seemed the shininess of Sydney had worn off.

I was 30 and decided I needed a change—not just a haircut or a new dress—a geographical one. So, I left Sydney full of faith and headed to the USA. It was here that the spell of LA took its hold of me. I was mesmerised, and to a degree, caught up in a lustful trance that lasted a decade.

I always knew I wasn't cut out for a corporate gig, and LA was perfect for nurturing my blue-sky thoughts. It was here in the city of angels that I realised that we all had wings and it was up to us to use them, and we were encouraged to do so. While I knew I was one of the hundreds of thousands of civilians that flocked to this west coast city, I was thrilled to be another number living in the land of opportunity. A place like no other where I was fuelled by ambition, possibility and lots of terrible filtered black coffee.

North America offered me something exciting and different that I yearned for. It pushed me outside my comfort zone while at the same time saturated me with new sights, smells and conversations.

TRAVEL has, and will always, seduce me. Movement and constant scenery changes fuel my life ride. It's kind of like blood pumping through my veins. But at the time, CAREER was my living force. It often fought with the second item on my list, which was LOVE. The two rallied against each other throughout my twenties and early thirties, jostling in and out of first place. Kind of like children squabbling over winning shotgun position in the car. Neither were ever ultimate winners though, as neither knew they needed to work together to bring about any kind of success.

CAREER's ambitious force would often win the prime seat at the wheel and LOVE rode in the back. The two would constantly nit-pick one another but neither could be at the driver's seat at the same time nor could they ride evenly alongside one another in the front. This symbiotic chaos seemed to exist for almost everyone I knew in LA. At the time, securing a successful long-term relationship in the city with someone worthy was a long shot just as much as it was for an actor to win a lead role in a union paying film. I was in the land of 'me' not 'we'.

Within a couple of months of landing in LA, I was offered the lead hosting role on an all-girl DIY makeover show for the LOGO network, which back then was primarily aimed at LGBTIQ viewers. This reinforced my decision that moving to Hollywood was the right one for me. I was able to dig up and create enough documentation to substantiate my application to secure an O1 'alien of extraordinary ability' working visa. Once I did, I promptly called LA home.

While that 'all-girl DIY home renovation series' never made it to the big screen, it was how I unearthed my passion for show development and script writing. I realised I enjoyed the creative aspect behind the camera rather than in front of it. So I began writing treatments and pitching my ideas with other producers. A DIY eco-series became my passion project and was thrilled when it was picked up by a production company who pitched it to the networks. Once I did that, though, I was at the mercy of Hollywood; I'd fallen hard and fast into the cliché LA producer bubble.

I learned quickly that it was all about playing the waiting game, which included the talk. The constant meetings. The constantly cancelled meetings. The booze-free lunches. The constant adulterous requests over the booze-free lunches.

I remember one entertainment lawyer even offered to pay my rent in exchange for dinner and a "catch up" once a week. It wasn't like I was completely unprepared for all the whack and wank of this town as I had come across my fair share of BS navigating my way through the media channels back home. But I'll never forget how many coincidences I had in those first few months of arriving in West Hollywood. Every time I came within a few feet of someone...anyone...they were quick to tell me all about themselves.

I must have reeked of fresh meat because people literally threw their business cards and resumes at me wherever I was. One time, I was standing at a traffic light, and a guy in a wheelchair talked me into sitting down and having a coffee with him to discuss his projects. As I walked home scratching my head about that guy, another one almost ran me off the footpath to throw me his headshot and contact details. Okay, I may not have been radiating actress vibes, but I don't think I fit the producer stereotype either. Yes sweetie, welcome to Hell-Ay!

I was naively surprised at how serendipitous it seemed that there was always a producer, writer, actor or director within a 20-foot radius of me. It obviously clicked not long after, but I'll always laugh at myself for orchestrating a new life in the worlds entertainment hive, then still be completely blown away every time I stumbled upon "industry peeps".

While I spent my days dreaming up TV projects and putting together development ideas I also did a little private cooking and catering on the side. My little business called Barbie Babes started off solely as a TV project with Aussie chicks serving typical Aussie BBQ all around the city. I soon realised it would actually work as a business venture and started catering events. It was fun, for a while, but was also demanding— moving a one-tonne stainless steel BBQ all around town isn't as sexy as it sounds!

For the most part, the business had pizzazz but lacked heart. Having been a vegetarian since I was fourteen years old, it was out of alignment with who I was and still am; that is, throwing down cheap steaks and snags didn't sit well with me at all. This became quite apparent when two of my friends and I were contestants on Season Three of the Food Network's 'The Great Food Truck Race' (TGFTR) a reality competition show where teams are given a budget and set challenges by the host, Tyler Florence, as they travel through different cities across the US.

I saw the ad on Craigslist, boldly applied, then was shocked, not to mention completely clueless, when we were selected to be on the show. We hadn't ever watched an episode and really weren't interested in winning a food truck. What we did desire were adventure and cash. We definitely nailed it with the adventure part, albeit only for a short time, but certainly not the latter. I struggled with purchasing supplies from the restaurant depot, which required us to select the cheapest minced meat blends and slaughtered sliced and diced cow in bulk.

So, of course, once we were off the show, my low-end-throw-down-BBQ-style evolved into high-end, sustainably-sourced creations with a strong vego theme. I felt I could only cook meat if I knew every single morsel and ligament would be sucked from the gristle by a hungry human. I loathed the idea that an animal's life was so haphazardly discarded without any real consideration or apathy for its life being brutally cut short.

What was quite amusing to us was when on the second challenge we were given the task to cook vegetarian food. Secretly, we laughed that we would kill it, without actually "killing it" that round. Little did we know that this now would kill us in the competition.

The way to win was through sales, and we were totally off the mark. We just weren't in it to win like the other teams who dreamed of owning and operating a food truck. But just as we decided to hand over our keys to keep another team in, we were informed we didn't make it to the next round. So, we said our farewells to the other teams and hot-footed it out of Arizona and back to LA. That's where our adventure ended but where I found my truth. From that day onwards, the Barbie Babes biz honoured its vegetarian roots.

The food truck experience was a real turning point for me (even a ten point one at that wheel) as it was one of only a few rare, awkward steps towards giving myself permission to stand up for my true message publicly. It was like I kind of got the balls to back myself and it was OK to be different, be my message, especially in business.

I settled back into everyday LA life, but while catering my good friend Michelle's kid's soiree in the Palisades, she offhandedly asked me if I ever wanted children. Without hesitation, I blurted out, "yes." Apparently, I was now on a roll with this honesty/living in alignment thing. I hadn't been that candid about my baby desire to someone before. It was like she tapped into my unconscious mind and could relate to what my heart really ached for. A brutal layer slayer, she had ripped off what I had bound myself so tight up in.

She asked, "Why don't you go home to Australia and focus on meeting someone?"

Australia? Oof! I wasn't ready to let go of LA nor would CAREER let go of it. At that time LOVE was, unfortunately, sitting next to my other life loves, TRAVEL and FRIENDS in the car who also had their own backseat battle of order. LOVE got drowned out amongst all their banter as it wasn't ready to truly be acknowledged.

My years in LA were big ones for personal growth, even though my sole focus for being there was work. Babies, children and family were so far outside the bubble I created for myself in the same way I had geographically put distance between Australia and me. In between TV production gigs that sucked up all my energy for months at a time, my days were filled with happy hours, 10am breakfast meetups with "potential collaborators" and late morning canyon hikes. A lifestyle that had no space for little people. My main priority was to be successful. I'm not really sure what that definition really represented back then, but I know for sure that success has a very different meaning to me all these years later.

While I also imagined and expected I'd always find an insanely wonderful human to live out the rest of my days with, that human never showed up. Or stayed. So the idea of having a family couldn't really ever become anything more than a silly made up movie in my mind because he didn't exist for me. And to be honest, because he wasn't there, kids just couldn't be either.

It didn't mean I didn't search for him. Whomever he was. As each birthday rolled into the next, the turning of a higher digit never sparked the idea to maybe ponder the number a little longer. I failed to notice I was getting old and never thought for a moment he wouldn't eventually show up.

While children weren't part of the picture in my early thirties, they were always unconsciously part of my grander life vision. Somehow, though, I failed to acknowledge the looming biological deadline creeping up on me.

Living in a place where Botox and big dreams turn back time and every man is a Peter Pan, ageing drifted through time just as each hour slid by sipping the next cocktail at another fancy rooftop bar. I hadn't had any luck in finding true love in LA so maybe Michelle was right, it would be smart to shift focus and throw out a line elsewhere.

I was 37 when LOVE finally kicked CAREER out of the front seat. LOVE finally had all the power. I only realised this when James managed to stir my hot pot of emotions. He was a straight-laced and pretty boy architect that I dated for six months just before the girls and I signed on to do TGFTR. We met through an online dating site and even though it was only a few weeks before my summer trip back to Australia, I caught up with him at a local bar. I was instantly attracted to him physically, and it helped that our banter could transcend time. Before we knew it, it was after midnight, and we were still completely enraptured in one another. It didn't take long then for us to be wrapped around one another.

I was the first woman he'd had a relationship with since his divorce the year before. He was a bit of a nerd and lived life playing it safe. I encouraged him to live a little by jumping on an Airbus and meeting me in Australia. At first, he declined, as it was far too radical to do that with someone he'd only known for a month. I shrugged it off and once I landed in Sydney, I headed to the Blue Mountains for my planned check out of life and fill up on a bunch of enriching nothingness and bowls of hearty vegetarian meals at the Vipassana Meditation Centre (Dhamma Bhumi) for ten long days.

Putting out the emotional trash while cutting out the noise seemed like a novelty and a grand way to offload some of the crap I had collected over the years. The word Vipassana means to 'see things as they really are' and apparently it works via osmosis too. Once the ten days of silence were over, I turned on my phone and to my surprise, there were a bunch of messages from the cutie-batootie draughtsman who was now desperate to buy a ticket to the land down under.

Clearly going off-grid was the way to shake up his heart. It gave him some quiet time and space so common sense could kick in. Once the idea had marinated, he too couldn't understand why he wouldn't bring his dorky butt down under.

Needless to say, James arrived in Sydney a month later on New Year's Eve. We were so blessed to be staying at my mate Steve's place who just so happened to have an apartment in Potts Point with a stunning uninterrupted view of the harbour bridge. Let's just say his adventure down under got off with an almighty bang. The New Year's fireworks display was great, too. It was a magical start to our week-long road trip up the coast to Noosa in Queensland.

I was in Australia for another six weeks once James left. When I did return to the US, we settled straight into an everyday relationship routine. I cooked dinner. He did the dishes. We did our laundry while we watched "our" TV shows together, and he managed them with the remote. I barked orders at him to turn it up, pause it, turn it down and rewind when I couldn't hear what they were saying. I'd say we were coasting along AOK until he stung me in the wee hours of the night with his poor bedside manner. While cradling me after we had completely ravished each other, he blurted out, "You'll make a wonderful wife to someone one day."

I knew we were comfortable with one another, but those words at 2 a.m. were way too close for comfort. They landed really hard. So I shook myself out of our embrace, got dressed and dashed out of there. This scene was eerily similar to the one I'd experienced nearly fifteen years earlier with Franz. I cried until the sun rose the next day. James and I never saw each other again as I didn't feel there was a reason to keep wasting time with someone I liked a lot but didn't love.

And as much as those words in that moment were incredibly hurtful, it was the reality jolt I needed. Coasting along was not going to give me what I wanted. So, it was a relief that finally, my tears were for something I wanted and not for something I didn't. The idea of MARRIAGE had secured a seat in the car and LOVE had its foot on the pedal and hands on the wheel.

# Chapter 3
# SHIPS - The Life Changing Three

*"A ship in port is safe, but that's not what ships are built for."*
*- John A Shedd, author. Popularised by Grace Hopper, computer*
*scientist and badass naval woman*

WHILE *I* NEVER WANTED TO get married or have children in my twenties, I did grow up always thinking I'd get married and have a family because that's what I believed relationships evolved into. I envisioned wearing the white dress and standing alongside a man who was mesmerised by me and me captivated by him. Having just turned forty, I was upset as to how I got here without a child, a fiancé, marriage or divorce. My inner dialogue somehow always circled back to present me with the idea that I was possibly not worthy to have all things. Or maybe I've been closed off from allowing them to enter into my life. I questioned if I had ever been truly living, or living like James and playing it too safe.

I'm not sure if divorce was a goal worth achieving, but, I mean, even James had that one on his list. I didn't and could only put it down to the fact that I didn't settle or I wasn't marriageable. Either way, it didn't matter. I was where I was and my present state had me swiftly shift gears from living life 'In Time' to one that lived 'Through Time'.

If you're not familiar with this reference, it stems from Neuro- Linguistic Programming (NLP) which implies there are two types of people when it comes to time. 'In Time' and 'Through Time' people. An 'In Time' person is someone who lives more in the moment, keeps options open and rolls with whatever happens. There's no internal clock ticking away and there tends to be no planning ahead. A 'Through Time' person is more conscious of the value of time and is therefore good at planning, meeting deadlines and showing up on time.

In my twenties, I was a dedicated 'Through Time' person who worked with time to get a degree and carve out a career. However, when I moved to LA I somehow fell into being an 'In Time' person. I guess my career path in Australia was served to me in bite-sized chunks, and I could chew at them without choking. But in LA, it was like I catapulted myself to a mountaintop and even though I was close to touching the moon, the sky was endless, which meant so too were the possibilities. With hundreds of thousands of stars twinkling before my eyes it was just too overwhelming. It was easier to aim for my own targets. Ones where I could keep shifting the goalposts. Basically, ones that were achievable in their or my, own convenient time.

Clearly, time had caught up with me; it was time to get back on track and live life 'Through Time', especially, when time wasn't ever slowing down, and my fertility window was steadily winding up.

I had wasted enough time in life staying in relationSHIPS with the wrong men, holding onto exhausting friendSHIPS and expecting combined business and personal partnerSHIPS to actually work.

I had to let many SHIPS sail.

Apart from my brief mateSHIP with James, there are three main relationSHIPS worthy of a mention that shaped my life story up until now.

## BIG LOVE NUMBER 1 – Eternally Yours For Now

When I was eighteen years old, while I was travelling around London, I bought my very first boyfriend, Franz, a professional athlete at the time, a gold ring for his 21st birthday. I had it scribed with the words "Eternally Yours, Hayley". I was eighteen! It was fair to say I was besotted with this blonde-haired, blue-eyed beast of a human; I didn't care that that gold ring cost me my return ticket back to Australia. While my physical self was travelling about in London, my brain and heart were dancing around to their very own beat.

Franz was my BIG LOVE #1 and I had been crushing on him for two years before he actually knew I existed. He had come on my radar when I ventured out to a local sports event with my friend Kerry to watch her brother compete in a local athletics competition. One look at Franz as he brushed past me on the street and my heart was completely stolen.

Nearly two years later, I was working full-time in a photographic store saving my pennies for my 'travel the world' savings account. I actually didn't know what I wanted to do with my life beyond travel. Travel seemed to romance my soul. Just thinking about flying somewhere foreign gave me butterflies and my eyes sparkled for it. Working a nine- to-fiver was my way to grow wings as travelling required lots of dollars.

One groundhog working day, I saw Franz standing at the counter. He had come in to drop off a roll of film for processing, and I went so weak in the knees I could barely shuffle my way over to assist him. Avoiding eye contact and barely able to stutter out some words, I somehow managed to ask him for his name, address and phone number, which I filled in on the customer processing docket before he even responded.

Knowing when he was likely to be back to collect his pictures was an important detail, too. He had no idea who I was, which in that moment I was thankful for. Those were the days when I didn't wear any makeup other than some foundation to blot out a few pesky pimples, which I always managed to sculpt into embarrassing moon craters across my forehead.

I never really made much effort in the mornings to look hot for work, but after that visit, I tried to put my best face forward. While I couldn't titivate my oversized uniform, I knew I'd feel a million bucks giving some attention to my frazzled mane and brightening up my pale face with some lippy, mascara and a puff of bronzing powder.

Unfortunately, Franz didn't return on the day he specified to collect his packet of photos, which I had even naughtily discounted. His pics sat in the draw for the following two weeks, which just so happened to be my final two at that store location. I had taken a last-minute transfer to the city due to staff changes and in doing so, not only lost my direct physical access to Franz but also my sneaky fly on the wall opportunity to peek into his life.

I presumed he never returned because he was somewhere on the other side of the globe competing in another competition and immortalising more memories on more Kodak 35mm film. From inside my fluorescent work-box stationed inside a shopping mall where I was surrounded by cameras and photo machinery, I could only fantasize about the feeling of flying so free.

While I knew being privy to seeing his life in pictures had subtle characteristics of what's termed a stage-five-clinger these days, I couldn't wait to share my jaw-droppingly awesome news about his store visit with my friend Kerry. She then relayed this news to her brother, who then told Franz that a girl in the local photo shop had a major crush on him and had an all access pass to his photos. I didn't dare share that I had made doubles of the ones I liked and kept them for myself.

With Facebook and Google such an open platform giving gawking privileges into anyone's bubble these days, my crazed crush behaviour wouldn't even push an eyebrow hair out of place of any millennial. Back in 1992 however, I had complete access and a preview into people's private and social lives that kids today have free reign to copy, share, manipulate and even sell.

Unrestricted photo access was the best perk of the job. Not that many people's images sent me into a tizz like Franz's did. Yes, there was a tonne of weird shit that came through that we had to develop, colour correct and sort through. One of the most fun things to do was to put the naughtiest ones on top, so when the customer returned to pick up their pack you'd show them the top image to confirm the order was theirs. It was the highlight of our day "outing" people so to speak and witnessing their red faces in those moments. Amateur nude modelling photo shoots was very popular!

When Franz got word that "Photoshop girl" had a crush on him, he took it upon himself to get in touch with me for a chat followed by a visit to meet me in person while I was working at my new store in Perth's Hay Street Mall.

He and a friend dropped by to suss me out, which must have gone okay as I secured a date for that following Friday night. I passed that test, too, which was the catalyst of a two-year long-distance relationship. It took this everyday shop girl out of Gosnells and catapulted her to official WAG* status.

*An urban acronym for the 'wives and girlfriends' of sportsmen (originally footy players). Basically 'his' glorified accessory cheering on the sidelines or in the grandstands of sporting matches.

Once we finally got together, I just thought Franz and I would always 'be' and that we would one day have a bunch of mini Franz's running about.

He was my taste of first love. Perhaps at the time that also included visions of a five-tiered cake and a white poodle dress. Although give me some credit, I wasn't deluded enough to create a glory box full of outdated crap for our future home or a vision board projecting our perfect life.

One of our most glorious moments was in Vail, Colorado, while he was doing high altitude training. After cavorting around London with a couple of girlfriends for a few months, I flew to the US to spend a couple of weeks with him. As the only WAG unofficially on tour, I was swiftly relegated to kitchen and cleaning duties. It was hardly glamorous but it gave me something to do while the team was out training for up to eight hours a day.

As each day rolled into the next, I could see where and how I fitted into this picture. Reality really kicked me in the guts on the eve of his 21st birthday, when I discovered he had been unfaithful since I had last seen him a few months prior in the Netherlands. Completely blind- sighted, I picked up the gifts I had for him and threw them at him. Remember that ring I had scribed for him in London? Well, it was now firmly planted on the side of his head from an almighty baseball pitch from across the room. It left a nasty bump and seemed to be the only mark I left on him. It was the least I could do.

Even though I wouldn't see him for another four years, he managed to keep me hanging on the line. This was despite him travelling the globe, dating other women and cutting out on communications for six months at a time.

When an overseas number showed up on my phone, I would always pick it up. I always knew when it was him. He was a habitual creature calling me at any hour because he was too lazy to figure out the time difference. His calls would come from exciting places all over the planet where he was either training or competing. I still held a flickering flame for him and hoped he had one for me. After all, why else was he calling me?

In late 1998, Franz phoned me from France and told me he wanted to come and see me. Be with me, because I was the girl that was always there for him. About a week later, at the end of October, he arrived at my doorstep in Sydney. This just so happened to be my birthday week and my final weeks of university.

I was nervous and excited that this man had finally awoken and was coming to get me. Having not seen him in so long, our first initial hello was a little awkward. So much had happened in those years prior so there was a lot of conversation to be had. But he just marched through my doors with his ego leading the charge. His behaviour was very distant from the moment we set eyes on one another, but I overlooked this, and many other of his selfish behaviours, as deep down I was hoping he'd finally see that I was 'the one'. After enjoying a late afternoon birthday romp together, we got up and began dressing for dinner. In the midst of the 'getting dressed chaos', and me mid-button on my shirt, he blurted out the words, "I don't love you."

These four single syllables shot me in my knee caps and ricocheted through my heart.

I rushed to the kitchen, where Kim, who was my roommate at the time, was making herself dinner and thrust myself into her arms. I sobbed for perhaps ninety seconds and then said, "No it's my birthday and I'm going to dinner."

Thankfully, a knock at the door tore through the house to shake up the mood and slice through the awkwardness. It was Sven, Franz's best buddy who was joining us for dinner.

I relied on him to deflect the pain of my shattered heart and enhance the evening atmosphere. To add some salt on my wound, though, the bastard Franz didn't even pick up my dinner bill. He left for Noosa, Queensland, the following morning and I handed him his shoes and told him to never, ever contact me ever again.

Our eternal flame had finally burned out.

Franz eventually got married and had four little blue-eyed creatures with somebody else, so needless to say when he contacted me eleven years later I was shocked. He said that he had seen me on Facebook and really wanted to reach out but wasn't sure if I'd respond—that I had made it very clear that day when I farewelled him there was never to be any contact again.

Thankfully, time does heal shattered dreams. In fact, by that point he was so far in my past, he was barely a blurry figure in my rear vision mirror.

We caught up a few times for drinks in Los Angeles, which would often turn into confession sessions. On one occasion, he told me I was his greatest regret. Thankfully, he wasn't mine. Sitting opposite First-Love-Franz, the man who held my heart for eight entire years, went on to reveal that he and his wife were heading for Doomsville. Karma, finally? Or perhaps had he finally realised that I was, and have always been, 'the one'—like Camilla to Prince Charles?

Oh, hell no. Well, not for me at least. We were two completely different people having had lived completely different lives. Sure, more than a decade earlier I was beside myself in a world of confusion and torment, but I was also thankful he left my world when he did. He had finally set me free, or so I thought at the time; ultimately, it was me that had let go.

While we sat there at a small bustling Santa Monica pub, he continued to divulge a year or two of his relationship sludge as I silently sipped my beer; my mind wandered off creating a series of future scenarios.

Scenario One: Franz and I rewind twenty years and pick up where we left off. Face squishes up. Nope! I definitely don't want to go back to my twenties to be this guy's doormat.

Scenario Two: I relocate back to Australia, after Franz and his wife call it quits. Then he and I move into a tiny two bedroom apartment, and I become the other woman his four children aged three to thirteen hate for just being alive.

Scenario Three: He gives up his life in Australia to be with me in the US. I would then become a therapist to an overweight, middle-aged and worn-down man who has rebounded. I would still be 'that' other woman to his four kids: the one who stole their daddy and put a crapload of ocean between them.

Still in denial about my ageing child-bearing countdown, taking on a freshly separated man with four beasties couldn't evoke even the faintest of twitches from either of my shrivelling ovaries. I also knew that he was about to be snipped, so it was a dead end in every way. I wasn't at all attracted to him anymore, anyway. He didn't look well at all and was thankful I danced down a different road.

Still, that relationship shaped me as a person, and our initial bust up contributed to my dedicated pursuit of a career in the media. It pushed me all the way through university and a relocation from Perth to the television hub and bright lights of Sydney. While we were only officially a couple for two years, that break-up obliterated my naive heart into thousands of tiny pieces and consumed me long after he was gone. Franz, and the residual pain from that relationship, unfortunately, played a pivotal role in turning my bright starry-eyed marriage dream into Kryptonite.

## BIG LOVE NUMBER 2 - SLAP OF THE GHOST
### 'A mis-wired and mis-fired gutsy love'

I was 29. He was 31. I lived in Sydney. He bunked in Brisbane. His name was Trey and from the moment I met him I couldn't imagine not wheeling our love into a nursing home together. We were brought together by a mutual friend who thought I was the perfect purl to follow his knitting stitch. All she told me about him was that he was a tall, blonde, athletic man who worked in property development with his family and was single, but apparently, she pumped me up pretty good.

In the heat of Australia's blistering summer, he happened to be hanging beachside in Sydney, so contacted me to see if I lived up to the hype. A sauvignon blanc was the perfect way to reel me in and cool me down on this hot 30 odd degree January day. Within hours of his call, I was at a nearby pub sitting opposite him. Not only was he two years older than me, he was also two feet taller. A former Olympic sportsman, charming and sophisticated—the heat of the day was replaced by me being on heat.

I was instantly attracted to him and we fell swiftly into a whirlwind affair. The type that sent blood gushing through my veins and electricity through every cell of my being. These signs reinforced the idea that he and I were a 'we' and meant to be forever and ever.

It was the second time in my life that I'd ever experienced the rush of Zsa Zsa Zsu. These three Z's are words that capture the zing between two people that are unique and indescribable to each of us. It's the knowledge that someone gets you and has got you. It's the butterflies, the stomach knot, nervous energy, the 'I can't get enough of you now' electricity. You'd be familiar with this term if you're a Sex and the City fan. Carrie used it in an episode to explain that feeling when you first meet and fall in love with 'the one'.

Trey continued to travel the nine hundred kilometres (or 450 or so odd miles) south to spend time with me and I would head north to do the same. We enjoyed luscious weekends enjoying all the hot spots around each other's cities. This man had my heart. I felt safe and invincible when he was around. If I dropped a stitch this man would catch it. We both focused on work during the week but the weekends were ours to keep weaving ourselves together.

However...after months of euphoria, he flew down one weekend and came by my place before telling me he was going to hang with his mates for a while. When the day turned to night and he still wasn't back, I began texting and calling to see what was up. He didn't return my calls that evening. Or the entire next day or the one after that. He just vanished. No explanation. The heartbreaking reality was—he ghosted on me. It was a jaw slapping wakeup call that what I thought was happening between us was clearly not reciprocated.

My gut had guided me to LOVE. It was an illusion put on not by The Magic Castle but The Magic Asshole. I couldn't fathom how this could be. It made no sense and spiralled me into a grey 'I don't know' fog that followed me about for almost a year. I was so stripped of emotion that my dear friend Amy pulled me aside and told me how worried she was about me. She even booked me in for spiritual and emotional help with a therapist. I was unaware that the grey numbness was seeping out of me, staining everyone and everything I came into contact with.

I explained to the therapist that in my mind, I was sitting high on a branch up in the sky and could see myself below functioning in this grey cloud. But there was an end to it. I mean, the only way to get through the pain of this loss was to get through it. I knew I would, and time in this instance was what I had on my side.

Of course, nine months later, once I could finally see hues of blue, Trey came to town and contacted me to catch up for a drink. After throwing a shot of vodka courage down my throat, I drove to the other side of town to see him. My mission was to uncover the clues that I must have missed leading up to his vanishing act.

I arrived at the bar in Bondi to a warm and happy embrace and a bottle of Pinot Gris. I, on the other hand, was a cocktail of Absolut confusion. After an hour of superficial chit-chat and two bottles down, he invited me up to his hotel. I thought now was my chance to pounce and strip him of information as to why he split without a word.

He, on the other hand, saw this as an opportunity to pounce and strip me naked. Refusing to divulge anything, opting to suck my face off and tear at my clothes like a savage instead. Like some animalistic skin on skin reconciliation action was going to feed my soul.

I refused. He erupted.

I kept asking him why he left and where he'd been, but the alcoholic fumes only fuelled his rage. Next thing he was pushing me into my car demanding I leave. Both shaken and stirred by his frenzied state and knowing I was over the legal limit for driving, I reluctantly moved the car around the corner, pulled over and snoozed off his serving of vitriol.

While I never got the answers I was hoping for, I realised that night he couldn't have been 'the one'. Our happiest times together were always when Glenfiddich, Belvedere and Penfolds joined us. My long unanswered questions were finally resolved as it was clear as day that night.

Unfortunately, it also reinforced the belief that my gut was never to be trusted, which for me was the foundation LOVE was built on and where Zsa Zsa Zsu grew.

## BIG LOVE NUMBER 3 - LIFE LOVE NOT LOVE LIFE

It was quite fitting that only a short time after James, the pretty boy architect, told me I'd make a great wife for someone else, that I met Ian. This man grabbed the driving wheel of my life and within weeks we became instantly entwined. An Aussie bloke living in LA, he was so down to earth. Real. Smart. Super cute and the third man I dated in 20 years that had 'ring on finger' potential. I didn't see him as my part-time lover; he was the whole kit n caboodle. I was smitten with us. This. Whatever he and I were, I believed we had the potential to be that. Together.

He came in a very different package to other men I had been dating in LA—he was an Aussie. I figured having been scorched by my most notable relationships one and two, that at 37 I needed to take a very different approach with this one. So, I locked my heart away and had my brain and body lead the charge. While I mentally and physically showed up, I really wanted my emotions to join in last. History had shown me that the Zsa Zsa Zsu could not be trusted in making these kinds of decisions. And after my massive slap in the face with Trey the Ghoster, there was no way I was allowing my heart or gut guide me to LOVE.

Ian knew he arrived in my world when I wasn't representing myself at my best. I was jaded in life and love. Tired. Even a little lost. He could feel it more than he could see it. He took my hand anyway. He was the brimming warm, sweet brewed pot of tea to my empty teacup.

We did have a couple of big obstacles to get through first. One was a massive singles party that I was hosting with a couple of friends just a couple of weeks after we met. Although my friends and I seemed to date a fair bit, we also always appeared to be single. Taking matters into our own hands, we decided to host a Christmas/holiday singles martini soiree at a mutual friend's home in Culver City. It was going to be the holiday event of all events to kiss the year goodbye, and fingers crossed, have a few people kissing each other's faces too.

It was an intimidating prospect for Ian, who had swiftly thrown his heart at me. But with the party date approaching fast, and my commitment to it first and foremost, I could only juggle it like a hot potato. We were expecting one hundred single guests to show up and always the faithful girl, I was totally focused on making it a success.

That Saturday night in December rolled around fast, and while we were still preparing, our guests started to fill the house one by one. I reluctantly invited Ian to the party as it seemed weird having just hooked up with him a couple of weeks earlier and now to have him come and mingle with all the other singles. I mean, it was awkward enough being one of the hosts while my status was transitioning from unattached to attached. Not to mention none of our partnered friends were invited. But he was adamant he wanted to be there. Probably to stake his claim in case any of the other stags tried to cut his lunch.

Our singles shindig was a huge hit and while I agreed the event went to plan, I didn't think we quite nailed it as no two individuals went home as a couple that night. Sure a few digits were exchanged, but only a select few filled their phones with names and numbers. Unlike a kids birthday party when everyone receives a candy bag on your way out, everyone else went home empty-handed.

It reminded me of the time I threw a singles dinner at my place when I was living in Brisbane back in 2002. My friend Jacqui and I invited a few guys we had dated but had no zing with, and a few of our single girlfriends over for a little mixer. As it turned out, the blokes were all hot for the same girl. That dinner was a total disaster, and I should have learned my lesson then: leave 'lurve' for the 'clurbs!' I guess I hoped LOVE would sweep me off my feet, so I was always creating ways for it to enter.

Our number two hurdle to love was crossing over the Chinese Wall. This is a term Ian introduced on our first date describing an ethical barrier within a business that creates conflicts of interest. Ian was, and still is, a serial internet entrepreneur and I was excited to learn from him; to pick his brain. At the time, I was bursting at the seams with business ideas and had been flogging one of them on and off for years. It was my passion project and it needed investment, experience and someone to believe in its vision as much as I did for it to lift off. I wanted it more than I wanted a man. However, if BUSINESS and LOVE came together as a package deal, well then, it was my ideal and ultimate 'SHIP'. And so a decision was made. We blew the top off the champagne bottle and climbed aboard.

I hadn't come across someone quite as dynamic as Ian whose ideas danced in a different paradigm. A risk taker. A mover and shaker. A man who could see the shiniest fish in a large frenzied school of baitfish. I told him about my ideas knowing he could make them roll. He really liked me but was hesitant about busting down the wall. He knew I was on my path with my ASPIRATIONS but something or someone had to fold for us to work. I begrudgingly threw down my round of cards pretty early on and then bottled up the resentment for doing so.

At the time, a life with Ian was never going to be one with an ordinary white picket fence. It was going to be a big life that a white picket fence couldn't fit around. He was the lead in his film and I filled the supporting role. His ideas were grandiose, often limitless, and he wasn't afraid to take a crack at trying them out. He was driven to minimally build a hundred million dollar global business that required a kaleidoscope of creative minds to carve out and bring it to its reality.

His galactic vision required lots of effort and sacrifice, which in a partnership can be detrimental. But the payoff would be worth it so we could then live a life on our terms. What that translated to was: work non-stop on developing his ideas and businesses and give up watching trashy TV, sleep-ins and long, boozy midweek brunches so we could do that anywhere around the globe in just a handful of years.

On the flip side, the relationship with Ian combined the things I treasured most—TRAVEL, LOVE, FRIENDS and BUSINESS. CAREER had reinvented itself under the guise of ENTREPRENEURSHIP which had totally seduced me. So here they all were my passions riding alongside each other together. I was especially euphoric knowing that there were a couple of spare seats saved for MARRIAGE and FAMILY. Miraculously, Ian had brought us all together in our life bus, of which he had a tight grip of the steering wheel.

His BUSINESS and my navigation skills took us all around the world. From our beloved LA across the USA, down to Barbados, across to Singapore, Hong Kong, Malaysia, Thailand, Bali, Australia, Europe, Dubai, Mexico, Central America, Aruba and back to our home in California.

We partied with a Punjabi family in Malaysia, spent a week in Puerto Vallarta Mexico for a festival of human spirit and entrepreneurial vision with 300 like-minded individuals, transformed our mindsets with Neuro-Linguistic Programming coaching in Bali, enjoyed some downtime, recalibration and brainstorming in Phuket and hit Costa Rica for adventure, inspiration and more entrepreneurial opportunities. With Ian, I felt like Julie Andrews on that hillside singing in complete joy with the world at my feet.

On the surface, I was living a big life... but more correctly, it was a big lie.

While these were life experiences I was grateful for and deeply cherished, over time their gloss wore off. They weren't implemented in the right order or united in their vision, and I wasn't happy.

We were always together, but we weren't functioning as a well-oiled machine should. It's like we were listening to the same song but tuning in on different frequencies. On the inside, LOVE wasn't truly being honoured and although I thought it was now leading the charge, BUSINESS had climbed into the passenger seat next to Ian, who was firmly driving this vehicle. Every idea was a new business opportunity and everyone else was given priority. I was ready to get married, but he was married to his businesses. I wanted to birth babies while he couldn't resist just birthing more businesses. I realised LOVE didn't stand a chance here, nor did MARRIAGE and FAMILY.

Early on we discussed having kids a few times but we weren't quite there. There was still so much we both wanted to do—places to see, opportunities to seek out. Besides, we hadn't really been together that long. I also knew he wasn't ready. I had every chance to call it quits only a year into our relationship while we were in Australia for what was supposed to be a short spin around trip that turned into a very, very long four-month stint, but didn't. I kept waiting.

As the writer and philosopher Alfred D. Souza apparently once said,

> *"For a long time, it had seemed to me that life was about to begin—real life. But there was always some obstacle in the way, something to be gotten through first, some unfinished business, time still to be served, or a debt to be paid.*
>
> *Then life would begin. At last, it dawned on me that these obstacles were my life."*

Fast forward a couple of years, our relationship continued to yo-yo in varying strengths. I needed some girlfriend time on the mothership (Australia) before our planned trip to Europe. We still had enough of a soft pulse to keep us ticking along, but I wasn't sure we had enough in our tanks to get us around seven countries unscathed, so I spent some time in Oz contemplating our future. He eventually jumped on the plane, or what I referred to as the defibrillator, to revive us; to keep us humming along.

We managed to band-aid us back together enough to slingshot it across to London. We figured, what didn't break us had made us stronger and we were ready to tear off our patches and resolve our issues. But sitting alongside one another in a confined space while he sped over European borders, and of course, with me navigating, had me verbally vomiting. Remember that frazzled road trip I mentioned earlier? Well, this is it.

By the time we pulled up at our hotel in France for the night, I was squealing at him, "You are a pig!" Sleep deprived, Ian was frustrated that

Siri, which was seriously dizzy, and I couldn't figure out how to locate our hotel on the block we were parked across from. It was 10 pm and pouring with rain.

Traffic was everywhere. We had just driven several hours and were incredibly frustrated, exhausted and over it. He lost his shit at me to try and figure it out. This blow out was not about driving directions, yet it was everything about driving directions. His hostility and my resentment were with us in the rental car, too. We were heading in different directions and we both knew it. Reality bites. And it hurt. Neither of us wanted to admit it so we didn't.

Once we landed back in LA, we quickly settled into the Silicon Beach lifestyle and our home became his start-up biz HQ with a turnstile of people and ideas at all hours. As part of his 'get fit' daily routine he'd head to an urban sweat lodge to ooze out his stress in an infrared bed, which only infuriated me.

Each morning, before his day got underway, he steamed his swimmers like a can of sardines. I fumed. I had made a claim on these baby makers and I needed them to not just be healthy, but alive and thriving. He was either blissfully unaware of the damage he was doing or maybe apathetic, refusing to acknowledge that when he got home my jumping up and down with arms flapping about wasn't justified. I wasn't engaging in a Richard Simmons fitness work out. It was 100% unadulterated "I'm going to kill you" rage.

That's the thing with dudes, they don't realise that turning up the body heat is a murderous event. I was so grateful he wasn't part of a MAMIL (middle aged men in lycra) cycling squad, spent any time in hot tubs or secreted out his toxins in daily baths. Still, I wanted every wriggler to receive a participation award and that meant they needed to, at the very least, make an appearance on race day. By that, I mean let the swimmers out of the gate and go at it, hell for leather to get to the finish line to claim the trophy which was one luscious egg.

As there was no official event ever planned between us, race day was always elusive. I was presumptuous in assuming we'd just be in the right window at the right time and we'd fall pregnant because that's how you have a baby right?!

Over those several months, I drank Ian's 'she'll be right, it's all cool' Kool-Aid but as it travelled to my digestive tract, it bubbled and boiled away with an excess amount of resentment that had burned through my stomach lining. I eventually spewed both up projectile style all over him. I had full-blown baby hunger that couldn't be contained. That's when he promptly got me a one-way ticket back to Australia for some more much-needed space from one another.

I didn't know it at the time, but it was the last time I was to ever step foot in our beachside pad. More time apart could not solve or resolve anything. Space was not going to bring me a baby. We were still one big gaping wound and we could not heal us.

Finally, Ian and my big life (lie) were done and I had no plan B.

## *Chapter 4*
# The Life Crash

*"I believe you can never fail in life or love. You just produce
results. It's up to you how you interpret those results."
- Karen Salmansohn, bestselling author of Think Happy*

SO THERE *I* NOW WAS, railroaded to singledom at the end of the world in
Albany, Western Australia. Ian and I didn't discuss our personal situation
as we didn't really know what banner "we" fell under. We both knew we
weren't right for one another. Heck, we'd become a miserable couple.
We were now living on different sides of the world; in fact, eighty-four
thousand Qantas' 787 frequent flyer points away from one another. It was
over, for us, and although it wasn't ideal, I continued working on one of
Ian's online businesses. It seemed to be a way for us to let go without the
shock of finality attached to it.

As uncomfortable as I was in my own skin, enduring the thick of
winter at my mother's house in the south west of WA also contributed to
my despair. I'm an ectothermic creature with a gypsy nature who relishes
warm climes. I snapped a bunch of 'ugly cry' selfies, so I could contemplate
the pain I was feeling. I was truly unhinged, feeling a combination of
disbelief that middle age had landed upon me, hurt that I wasn't enough
to be proposed to, grieving for the family I never got to have, stressed

by the climbing credit card debt and bewildered by what the hell I was now going to do with my life. I lost my home, boyfriend, security and my dream life in one foul swoop.

This wasn't my first big life slapdown; I'd had a few of those—minimally two each in the past couple of decades thus far. My Saturn Return (SR) twelve years ago was a doozy. If you dodged yours or haven't hitched your meltdown to any good reason yet, the SR may fit with this really shitty period in your life.

They are astrological phenomenons that descend upon us around the same point in our lives, at around 28-31 years of age. They're thought to occur when the planet Saturn returns to the same point in the sky it was in when you were born. This round trip "returns" signifying your transition into a new stage of life. It tends to be the time in life when you shed your childish skin and need to pull up your big girl knickers.

It's as frightening as hell as it typically brings a whole lot of chaos into your world with it, impacting relationships, having you question your career, friendships, home, sanity. Everything in life. So of course when my SR was in full swing, it made sense that at 30 years of age, I would turn my world upside down even more by moving to LA. Seemingly, I thought it'd be fun to treat myself with a scoop of double whammy with the wrath of Saturn Return on top.

This mega melt down however, came with my big, fat 4-0 fast approaching while I was perched on my gigantic life pile of poo at the bottom of the world with the chill of the Southern Ocean's icy Antarctic air infiltrating my entire core. I was on dead empty. And even though the breeze was cryopreserving my eggs for free, I struggled to find a silver lining. The only sounds that drowned out the chit-chat within were the ticking of two clocks: one, my pending fortieth birthday countdown, and two, the seconds lost on my fertility clock.

Each stroke was deafening and I was a fucking mess.

Oh, why oh why didn't I invest in icing my googie eggs before I got old? By my mid-thirties egg freezing was on trend. It was seen to be the golden ticket out of infertility, however, I naively never thought this was something I'd ever be implicated in. It was something others did. Not me. I ignored this SOS and now at my age, they were not only dying in startling numbers, but they were also less viable. Old eggs are far more susceptible to chromosomal abnormalities, just as I was to attracting the wrong men.

I knew the freezing egg process didn't necessarily guarantee me motherhood; it would, however, have guaranteed me hope. A future option. A fall-back plan. I knew that if I had frozen my eggs early enough, they would have had a better chance of one day being turned into a baby. In theory, I could use them any time, even in my sixties or seventies as I had learned in my research, the womb doesn't age. But I had blown this baby out of the frozen water. Literally!

A few days out from the big, fat erhem, I flew to Bali with my mum and bestie Shelley to spa, bar and massage away the pain of it all. I tried my best to keep it together for them but bottling it up didn't help. I needed to get every ounce of anger, sadness and hurt out. How wrong for a man to keep a woman on the line, screwing away her fertile window when he had no real intention of ever utilising it! Why the hell didn't he cut me loose and allow me the chance to find someone who actually wanted these things too? I felt like he used me to fuel his vehicle, to be his sidekick and didn't give a shit about filling up my tank!

Once I got over being mad at him, I turned the rage on myself. How could I let us drag on so long? How could I be so irresponsible to get myself here? Why didn't I take hold of the wheel years ago? Why didn't I take control of the nozzle and fill up my own tank? Right now, I am where I am because I got myself here. I realised he couldn't fill my emotional tank when he was running on empty too.

I stayed when I should have left. I put his wanting to have me in his life above me choosing me and what I wanted in my life. I truly was in deep caca with the hands of the biological clock ticking away.

I'd made it to thirty-nine years, fifty-one weeks, five days old and not even a divorce to tick off my list or number to add to a stat. As I gazed at my sad selfies through bloodshot eyes, I repeated to myself, "Oh yeah, I'm sure I'll make a wonderful wife to someone one day!"

# PART II

*I GET HOW I GOT* myself here, but why? I'm such a fuck up. Now look at me! Here I am frazzled on a plane on my way to meet a stranger to potentially make a baby with. Do I have a beacon on my forehead that sends out a signal stating my preference for guys who can't commit? Ones that don't want to put a ring on it? Or are my pheromones a total turn off to the opposite sex, in which case, I'm just not shaggable?

I always thought I would meet someone who would appreciate my simple girl ways dusted in Tinkerbell dreams and want to write them in the skies with me. I'm a dreamer, but not a princess. I've never been one to fuss about with makeup and clothes. I detest fashion shopping and certainly have never been a nightclub type. I'm much more the stay at home, girl next door type—cooking hearty meals in the comfort of my trackie dacks. While I'm a go-getter, I'm also much more of a home nester.

Sitting on the plane reflecting on my past relationship woes, I realised, perhaps that's the problem right there. I mean, I once invited a boyfriend who I had been with for a couple of months over to my place for dinner. I greeted him at the door dressed in my best Adidas sweats hollering, "Welcome, this is homey Hayley."

He looked surprised, and it wasn't in a 'wow' kind of way. I guess he was hoping for a little more effort from me in trying to impress him. I figured my cooking would do that, I guess. I grew up without a father and because Mum worked a full eight-hour day, she'd just be getting home to my brother and me when other families were already sitting around a table eating dinner together. So I began cooking super young. If Masterchef Junior was around in those days, I know I would have been a strong contender.

Our table was always set for three, and while I never felt there was ever a place setting missing, I wondered if this lack of older male presence was in reality, an invisible presence that played a much bigger role in my life.

*Chapter 5*

# The Back Story

*"A bend in the road is not the end of the road unless you fail to make the turn."*
*– author unknown*

MY FATHER SHOT HIMSELF IN the back of the head with a nail gun when I was four and a half years old, but his soul didn't depart this physical world until I was 25 years old. He lived out those years incapacitated in a nursing home while I was living out mine without him in our family picture.

We lived on a 10-acre property on the outskirts of Perth where my parents ran a wholesale fern nursery that my dad had built. We resided in a giant shed that was converted into a makeshift home. As far as my brother and I were concerned, our family life was normal and our 'casa garage' was too. However, life was anything but normal and Mum did her best to iron out the bumps so we kids didn't notice the rocky road she was travelling down.

Things had become so bad between my Dad and her that she moved the three of us to a nearby rental home. She was afraid of the man she once loved, and her gut instinct told her not to stay.

At six years old, my brother ran away from school early the day our dad attempted suicide and found him lying helpless in a pool of blood. So he did what any good Aussie kid would do—he ran to the kitchen, grabbed himself a glass of water and made a Vegemite sandwich. He handed them to him before running another kilometre to our home.

My mother called an ambulance the moment she saw him roll up on the front doorstep with our family dog; she just knew that my dad had done something and it wasn't good. It seemed to be his way of punishing himself or ending his torment over the violent physical abuse he had inflicted upon her only days earlier.

My brother and I were told it was an accident. That he had tripped over a piece of wood at our nursery. The word 'suicide' was too shocking to mention or swallow. A mishap, however, was much more bearable. We finally got the real scoop about "the" family catastrophe when we were teenagers.

Although Mum had fallen hard for him about a decade earlier, dad was apparently always a deeply troubled man. She didn't know why, and he certainly didn't show all his cards. She met him through her group of girlfriends, one of which dated a boy who was part of a local group of boys. Slowly the boy's group was infiltrated by all the girlfriends, which often brought them together socially for barbecues and camping weekends. These social gatherings were always boozy ones for the boys, which had my dad out drinking them more often than not.

Over time, Mum referred to him as "a constant disappointment" and distanced herself more and more from these get-togethers. Unfortunately, peering through her sober lens only reinforced her resentment towards him. As a result, they both distanced themselves emotionally from one another. Dad didn't talk about any of his woes; Mum didn't express her feelings. It wasn't that it was a closed topic of conversation, there just really was no conversation at all. Ever.

Dad ran his own roof contracting business. He was really good at building things but he was also good at breaking them. He traded his work days with drinking the daylight hours away at a few watering holes around the local area. More like a shadow in the dark than a father figure, he would stumble through the door to be greeted with cold dinners left on the dining room table. This was long after we babies were asleep and my mother was curled up in a slumber on her side of the bed. A mad reader, it was the heaviness of a page that weighed down her eyes and sent her off to the land of z's; it was no longer her tears or a heavy heart.

Dad would shuffle out the door in the mornings before any of us woke up to demand any attention from him. With alcohol consumption a daily ritual, it meant his libations expenditures ran high. He lost his paying clients and so, obviously, his income dried up. Of course, it was just a matter of time before his actions, or lack thereof, brought down our kingdom. First, his roofing business, followed by our family home and then his newer business, which was entwined with my mum's nursery.

One of the few stories Mum has of my father was when he painted his car to conceal his identity from the police. Apparently, he had lost his license for drunk driving but thought if he painted his car a different colour, he would still be able to drive to the pub under the radar. It seemed to work until the lid on the pressure cooker eventually blew off. A rise in a few degrees was all it took to push him over the edge and pull the trigger. He was only 32 years old.

With sightings of him around the house so rare, and being so young, I have no recollection of who he was. I actually don't have a single memory of him physically being in my life. He only exists in it because of photos. I don't know his mannerisms. His passions. His ambitions. What made him smile. What movies moved him. What bad dad jokes he collected and shared? What his favourite colour was or where his special place on earth was. He was never really talked about as I grew up either.

Not only was this story shrouded in shame, no one really knew how to broach it with us. It didn't help that my mother knew so little about him as well, but she also didn't dare investigate. Her marriage was a sham and keeping a united front while living separate lives under one roof was emotionally wearing and isolating. Blinded by love and reminiscent of the times which required keeping "it" together for the family (neighbours, friends, 'The Jones'), life went on, but just beneath the surface, the torment of this traumatic story lived on, too.

Waking up each day knowing he was in a nursing home being spoon fed was heartbreaking. As a young girl, I often cried for him. For his pain. His loss. Our loss. His struggle. Our struggle. It left a lingering sad cloud above us and my brother, mother and I grappled to shake it off. My mother often likened this calamitous situation to serving a jail sentence. Her misery bound up and oppressed in an emotional strait- jacket. She coped by merely existing. While there were many attempts early on, we didn't get any real relief or a real chance to start the healing process until he passed away twenty years later.

My mother did remarry briefly when I was eight years old, but that 'silverback' wasn't around long enough for us to watch him beating his chest. He wasn't a nice man. Rather an evil one, actually. As his stepchildren, we didn't exactly bond and he didn't hand us an olive branch.

Charmed by him and desperate to fall in love and share her life once again with someone, it took a little while for the cracks to show. Once he moved into our house, she realised she had opened her home and heart to not only Dr Jekyll but Mr Hyde too. Thankfully, she severed ties with both of them before they really settled into our lives. She once told me she had to marry him to get rid of him. I didn't understand what that meant back then but having stuck it out in manipulative and controlling relationships once too often, her words make so much more sense to me now.

Although she was bitten twice, it was a decade later when she thought she had finally found her life partner. Out of the personals from the local rag no less. Those were the good old days when it was embarrassing to publicly declare you were looking for love. Well, my school friends and I considered it so and would scoff at them after school while decimating a plateful of toasted sandwiches. And because the ad was printed in hard copy, it didn't vanish in a split second with one swipe. Nope, those ads inside newspapers landed on lawns of homes around a bunch of neighbourhoods and lived new lives at the bottom of grocery boxes, wrapped around flowers or at the foot of fireplaces for weeks, if not years.

His name was Des, and he moved into our place for a short time. My brother and I at this point were at the end of our teens and had mostly bounced from the nest, so this new male really didn't have an impact on us or our lives. To be honest, he didn't make a real impact on Mum either. After a decade together she called it quits because the relationship had lost its pulse.

I never knew what it was like to come from a "normal" family and have experienced a "normal" upbringing. As a child, I didn't get a choice in how ours looked. I thought of my mum as a mother/father combined role and to me, that was my idea of normal.

*Chapter 6*

# Nature or Nurture

*"I believe that there is a subtle magnetism in nature, which,
if we unconsciously yield to it, will direct us alright."*
*- Henry David Thoreau, author*

*"A man's character is his fate."*
*- Heraclitus, Greek philosopher*

WOULD *I* HAVE BEEN SO gung-ho in work and so pathetic in choosing love had I been blessed with a "normal" upbringing? By normal, I refer to what it looked like back in the day when it included a mum, dad and their kiddies living together under one roof. It ideally functioned with Dad going off to work eight hours a day, five days a week and Mum staying home to manage the house. Of course, this type of normal existed before The Brady Bunch TV show made blended families socially acceptable but what it lacked in its definition was "happily wasn't living under one roof". I think it's fair to say a fair chunk of the neighbours weren't the happy-go-lucky families, we saw beyond their manicured lawn and garden hedges.

With so little known about my father, I didn't have a whole lot to work with when it came to the DNA aspect. Was my Dad destined to hurt himself or be a chronic alcoholic? Did depression run through his veins? Was his struggle genetically linked or was it ignited by life stresses?

He was quite possibly mentally ill and went undiagnosed and untreated. Again, these years were the hush years where sensitive topics weren't discussed. Especially, not publicly or among friends.

As my guiding force, Professor Hawkins (whom I met along my 'rogue path") says, "The Aussie male is a different species to other males." They are most likely to frown upon any kind of counselling or psychological therapy. The 1960's was the 'be a man' era, which most wouldn't dare shed a tear, express his feelings to his woman, or sit with a stranger to unload. There was no such thing as a metrose ual and men didn t have man buns. Nope, dudes were more likely to beat their chests, hold their heads high and just get on with it. Talkin about it was not fly for a white guy or any guy for that matter!

Depression, sometimes referred to as clinical depression, is an illness and one that has genetic links. I recently cast my eyes over a study from last year that revealed teenagers who have a father living with clinical depression are at heightened risk of developing a mental health problem. My father's symptoms seemed consistent and were likely linked to a strain of the black dog. I concluded that it was very possible that it could have been passed down through the generation before him.

Word through the family grapevine was that one of my dad's relatives suicided due to alcohol and depression. While it hasn't been confirmed, and Mum never knew what family member it was and why perhaps there is a genetic link. But again, as it was pushed under the carpet, we have not to this day uncovered if this was true. Maybe alcoholism, depression, mental illness is deeply embedded in our stock? Or perhaps, having been exposed to suicide early on in his life, it was an influencing factor in him making that tragic decision?

Nature over nurture is a tricky one to really pinpoint due to how genes express themselves opposed to altering the genetic code itself. As I dug deeper, I found myself in the biology section of the library reading up on epigenetics. This is a field of study that looks beyond just accepting DNA as physical or mental traits being passed down through the generations. It looks at the link between the experiences and events that also impacted our grandparent's lives.

These experiences, such as surviving famines, can cause chemical "marks" to attach to genes and turn the activity of the genes on or off.

Basically, this means stress can alter cells, which are then passed down the family tree.

For example, the lifestyle of my great-grandmother when she was pregnant with my dad's father and the factors that influenced the health of her mind and her physical state. Depending on what was happening during the nine months my dad's father, my grandfather, was in his mother's womb, he may have been vulnerable to epigenetic events, which could have forever altered his sperm that in turn affected his offspring. In my case, my dad.

So maybe it's not a strain of bad eggs in my family line, but something that happened in my great-grandparent's lives that impacted my father's makeup, and it's not just hereditary or merely a 'mental thing', that is, buying into a story and then making that story his own. The mind is very powerful. Once you convincingly believe something it very likely becomes your reality.

Despite us all having cell altering powers, our age, lifestyle and the environment obviously also influence cell changes. So, I think it can be quite hard to pin down what really drives us. We are complex beings; some more than others.

While so much of who we are seems to be predetermined and influenced by major life events before we even poked our heads out of a womb, it also means the way we live our lives can affect our children's development and health as well our grandchildren's. I won't ever know how much of mine has been moulded by people of the past. I'll never really have access to that information and can only wonder where and how the little bits that make me up came to be what they are today.

It does, however, have me lament the nature versus nurture debate in relation to my failed relationship path. Is it due to nurture or lack thereof, or is there a biological link as to why it's not so easy for me to have that loving relationship I dream of?

When I look back on the trail of failed relationships that filled the gaps between my big love relationships like putty, I find an accumulation of narcissists: high-achieving senior managers, CEOs and professional sportsmen. It wasn't until a friend of mine pointed out the track of destruction left in my wake, that I saw the similarities. Before that, I figured it was due to the circles I moved in or because those were the dudes who actually made moves on me. I wasn't ever really good at showing my interest in the opposite sex; I basically had to be hit over the head to catch the signs.

Somehow, energetically, I attracted a certain type. Perhaps these men could sense the lack of daddy guidance in my life and therefore I was an easy target to emotionally control? Or did I unconsciously seek them out? Was it by nature or nurture that I am meant to be on this solo path? Having to grow up a lot earlier than other kids did suck. Coming home each day from school to a parentless house wasn't ideal. The emptiness was felt. Each day was just about making it to the next. Because of the financial pain my father got us into, it was one hell of a hole for my mother to dig us out of. Thank goodness she was born with a green thumb as gardening was her saviour.

For the most part, I wasn't really aware how hard it was. As a child, I just accepted what was. I had a working single mum. We always had a roof over our heads, food on the table and were surrounded by families of the same socioeconomic status. She didn't choose her situation but rolled with the punches. We may have lived in an average neighbourhood, but our house was in the fancier part of it, and she damn well made sure her garden was one of the best on the street.

Once I was old enough to understand that life choices could change my trajectory, I used our adversity to drive me and push me forward; to grab life and give it a good right swipe. My way forward wasn't necessarily easy, or in many cases, the most appropriate all the time, but I only knew what I knew, not what I didn't.

I've always been alerted of my family's history and how that may affect my future offspring, though. Would I have a child if there was a chance I'd pass some DNA malfunction onto them? I think as humans we all have favourable and not so favourable traits, but I think it's how a baby grows into their skin and less about what their cellular makeup is. It's how they manage challenges, what words they speak, and how safe and supported they feel.

It's the conditioning of those around them. Their immediate influences. People. Role models. Beliefs and rules imposed upon them on a macro and micro level. Their language and that of those around them.

I was shaped to value things, work hard and want more for myself; and to be mindful. If anything, my childhood and the man I never got to know played a large role in who I am today; it has given me the chutzpah, intestinal fortitude and wide lens to how I view this world. If anything, I hope I can pass a scratch of that along to the little person I'll be blessed to guide in this life.

## Education/Career

I was an average student who got average grades. High school wasn't my thing and when I was sixteen, I left to work full time in the photographic store I mentioned earlier. As devastating as breaking up with Franz was, it, along with the fact I was obsessed with travel, fortunately, inspired me to go back to school and finish my high school certificate.

Six months of travel, my first big break up, and a taste of a lifestyle bigger than I ever saw for myself, merged together to put me on a path that became my passion and obsession—sports journalism. A life that put me in front of hot men, required me to travel and it was a career. It was to be an extraordinary life and I was the one leading the charge.

I secured my year 12 certificate and then relocated to the east coast where I finished my bachelor's degree in journalism in Sydney. I felt I needed to be in the hub of media, and I couldn't do anything other than babble on about all things sports, news, and broadcasting. I volunteered at various media outlets wishing and hoping for a chance to get my foot in the door.

Not only did my Big Love Number One break up catapult CAREER to top dog in my value system, but it was also the 90s, a time when women really put their careers ahead of making babies. It seemed the city of Sydney manufactured this way of thinking and I was surrounded by Type-As. It was the norm and I willingly subscribed.

I got a great break when I went to SBS Sports and was able to put together VO packages for the nightly sports program. However, after a few months, the EP pulled me into his office and told me I'd never make it as a sports reporter or news reader as I looked far too young. What was so funny was just a few years later when working for Channel Ten's kids show, Totally Wild, I was filming a story about an up-and-coming soccer superstar. Just as I was wrapping on the story, the team manager came out to thank me and shake my hand for interviewing his player. I was shocked when I realised it was the former EP of the sports department who told me I wouldn't make it on TV.

I was 19 when I decided I wanted to work in the television industry. I was 25 when I finally landed a full-time gig with a national broadcaster as an assistant. I got that job by photocopying all my rejection letters and binding them together into what looked like a long Hollywood script. I figured this impressively bound bundle of no's was proof of my unwavering determination to work in the industry. I had access into the network as I had been working as a night time sports logger and took it upon myself to hunt down the Head of the Network and hand him my book of knockdowns.

After about 20 minutes of wandering about, I stumbled into him just as he was walking into another meeting. I introduced myself and thankfully he knew who I was. Mainly because he had rejected me so many times. He sat me down and then looked through the letters of which I had placed several of his on top. Two weeks later, I received a phone call and was offered a PA (production assistant) position with the network. My career in telly had officially begun.

Now sitting on this plane looking back, history has shown me that if I truly wanted something I could figure out a way to make it happen. Maybe having to work for everything from such a young age is what has given me a sprinkle of fearlessness to do so. I'm not sure how the next few hours will unfold, but what I do know is that I managed to untangle myself enough to get me here. I feel like a Rubik's cube that's managed to get all nine coloured blocks on one side to match green. And that means GO.

*Chapter 7*

# Pull the Ex Ripcord

*"It's not how you win or lose, it's how you place the blame."*
*- Ralph Kiner, baseball slugger*

THERE WAS A RIGHT FOOT *in, then it was out again. Then a hand in and then a hand out. This familiar nursery rhyme seemed to sum up my relationship. It included some hokey pokey, some shaking it about but instead of finally jumping ALL in...he turned himself around and flew away.*

Wasted Years Dancing the Hokey Pokey Despite slowly driving a knife into our intimate relationship, Ian and I did our best to navigate the complexities that go with a work/ex-partner relationship. During our three year relationship, we were more off than on anyways. Cold than hot. Closed than open. It seems to be a theme in my life that I keep hoping 'the one' will change; that we will get better together and our history will etch a blueprint that we can just keep ourselves attached to. To accept that a hard relationship is normal and get on with life.

For whatever reason, though, if a relationship isn't working, I will keep adding more air to it before driving a pin in it and slashing it so severely that there would be no way to put it back together again.

Stupidly, I often stash relationships in the fridge to chill out over months and sometimes years, hoping they'll retain some viability long after their healthy shelf life.

We knew, for the most part, we couldn't figure us out, but Ian loathed goodbyes and would do anything from entirely waving me farewell. I knew that by calling it a day, I'd be giving up my chance of motherhood. He put one foot in. He took it out again. He never put both in at the same time. I remained hopeful that one day he would and we could dance the Hokey Pokey with our kids.

Instead, I sang and danced along to that nursery rhyme for a year or two longer than I should have. Our relationship had stretched out long after its use by date. My crucial baby window was compromised by me not deeply acknowledging that time waits for no-one.

John Lyndsay Mayger (JLM) had seen this same story play out over decades as he tended to his donor role. JLM is a known AI donor for mostly lesbian couples and the biological father of 20+ little kids aged 1 to 14 years old. However, he was an unknown IVF donor between 1978-79, so actually doesn't know how many adults out there share his DNA.

JLM told me he heard countless stories of women who "had wasted their life on some male who says, 'Yeah, yeah, we'll just get the house and our careers settled and then we'll have a family,' but then at 37, says, 'No, I've changed my mind. I don't want kids, we're happy as we are and I just want to continue going along as we are.' The woman says, 'Yeah, but I want a family and you promised me that one day we'll have it.' Eventually, she pisses him off, then looks around and at 37 has to try and find somebody else. She then realises it's really hard to find someone in the marriage market in a short time frame because the biological clock is ticking."

I agree with JLM whose sound advice to women is, "At that age, you can't afford to muck around on dating sites, you've got to go straight to the sperm. Cut out the middleman!"

There's no doubt bringing a child into a relationship adds another dimension too; one that no-one can prepare for. Once bubs arrives, all the stuff between couples that's been stowed away for years eventually rises to the surface. Then that crap reaches a whole other level when it's combined with sleep deprivation.

While it was a long drawn out demise for Ian and I, mainly due to our work ties, thankfully he finally met someone else. He needed her. I needed her. We both needed something or someone outside of us to end us. Turns out she was the oxygen mask we both desperately needed independently of one another to revive ourselves. Let's sing this last line together: "And that's what it's all about!"

*"Free at last! Free at last! Thank God Almighty, we are free at last!"*
*- Martin Luther King Jr*

With Ian attending to blooms elsewhere, I truly felt free to explore other family options available to me outside the traditional landscape.

Until I confronted these thoughts that he and I were done, I was never in a fertile state. Energetically, I was holding myself back and my womb wasn't going to compromise itself for the wrong energetic combination. This isn't just new age thinking; our nervous, endocrine, and immune systems are actually so intimately entwined that they each affect the other.

I read somewhere that they're influenced by every thought we think and every emotion we feel and are constantly processing our thoughts, beliefs, feelings, as well as real-time images and dream sequences. These fine-tuned systems make up a larger one, which operates symbiotically impacting what type and how hormonal, chemical, neurological and muscular responses are made.

The combination of uncertain self-worth messages and limiting thoughts of what a woman thinks she wants can cause obstacles between her and the baby she so desires. This conflicting dialogue can throw off the delicately balanced hormonal system involved in reproduction, so clearing out the crap is essential to make way for good baby-making juju.

I finally returned to LA to collect all my belongings two years after Ian and I had completely flatlined. It was an emotionally hard return trip for me to make. I was scooped up by a friend at LAX then remained holed up in her nest for the following two days. Her apartment, located on a busy Culver City street, vibrated with every passing vehicle. I parked myself on her large balcony, so the traffic trauma could reverberate through my entire body while I inhaled a steady supply of smoggy LA air. As my compass reset itself to the familiarity of my former life, cold pressed turmeric and ginger shots did their best to counteract the life (time) change.

Once out of my jetlag stupor, I Ubered over to the Public Storage to finally face my decade of stuff. I collected the key from the front office and manoeuvred my way through the enormous maze to find the unit Ian had relocated my belongings for me to collect during my visit. The square piece of cement wasn't the warm, welcoming home I had left. It was neutral ground, though. A little cold. Detached and final. I unlocked the padlock and rolled the door up. There it was; the end of the end in one fifteen foot square cubicle. A barbed wire saliva ball gathered at the back of my throat shredding my flesh as it headed south at the same speed as the dropping ball at Times Square on New Year's Eve. There weren't any cheers, just a whole lot of tears.

My salty eyes scanned my scattered belongings. I was happy to reunite with some of it; the rest I was burdened by. My collection of life things had become a massive pain in my arse but the mammoth task of sifting through my once prized possessions had to begin.

It took me two days to decide what was worthy of being jammed into two extra-large battered suitcases and travelling ten thousand miles, and what wasn't. A dress I wore to Donatella Versace's birthday party in Beverly Hills. A gown worn once for a G'day LA event. My teeny tiny shorts I wore for playing beach volleyball on Venice Beach. There's no way one leg would squeeze into them now! Of course, there was a box of Barbie Babe's bikinis and tees. Oh, and my fave bomber jacket I had picked up in a second-hand store in a backend street in New York. Memories flooded back as I wrestled with farewelling them. Some I knew would have a new life with someone else, just as I would, once I cut this cord for good.

Now there was no more unfinished business or lingering hope for not only us but for my life in LA. It was the end of an era. It was another beginning of who I was to become. It was further reinforcement that we were completely done. Just as Carrie barked at Big in an episode of SATC (Sex and the City) that they were "so over" they needed another word for over, Ian and I had needed one for 'done'.

Unlike many couples who live out of one another's pockets, Ian and I never shared a bank account. Other than our emotions, access to some business files and a few material items, we were not entwined by any other means. Our break-up was ostensibly clean.

Once our ties were severed, I was able to truly follow my own heart and thoughts. His opinions and persuasive thoughts no longer impacted the decisions I needed to make. Even though I'm an expert in failed relationships with a stack of irrational self-help internal voices to assist in making shitty decisions, I was, fortunately, able to make at least one smart, swift and conscious decision: to limit indulging myself with sitting in my poo pile for too long. Been there. Done that.

I was now a 100 per cent, emotionally available, unattached middle-aged woman with an almighty goal to achieve, of which, at this point in time, I had no idea how the hell I was going to make happen. It was clear I had to get creative or become more open-minded about taking the steps to move forward as a single woman who now wanted to be a mother more than ever. Before I put a plan in motion though, I thought I had to resolve my why for wanting this. Why did I want a child? At 41, what was my drive now? While I didn't consider myself to be maternal, I always believed I'd one day be a mother. I just know I was meant to be one. Through every cell in my body, this I knew for sure.

My hurdle was that I wholeheartedly believed and wanted to conceive a child with the man of my dreams. Without him, how could I become a mum? I had been mulling over this realisation for over a year while for the most part, keeping out of sight in Australia while trying to figure it out.

When I was with First-Love-Franz I thought it would just be there for us. I thought Trey-The-Ghoster and I would hop to it. And with Hokey-Pokey-Ian, I figured it made sense. It was the natural relationship progression.

As I contemplated, it dawned on me that I didn't need to explain or convince myself or anyone my why. I felt my why.

# Chapter 8
# Sista's Without Misters

*"Help one another, is part of the religion of our sisterhood."*
*- Louisa May Alcott, novelist and poet*

I REACHED OUT TO A couple of my girlfriends who had already travelled down the motherhood path solo. They had to shift their perceptions of how life should be and how life actually is. They made hard life-changing decisions and thankfully, they succeeded.

Carmen, a good friend and former roommate of mine, had also kept a low profile while she set out on her path to pregnancy. It was a long, tumultuous four-and-a-half years that had her move through round after brutal round of IVF. Thankfully, her perseverance and high emotional tolerance brought her a gorgeous little girl. It wasn't without a lot of frustration, heartache and a good chunk of cashola though.

It was only during her mid-thirties that she started to think about children. At the time she still considered it a 'one day' type of thing. Something that would happen down the track with someone.

Like many of us, she didn't consciously base having kids on any specific predetermined terms or a timeframe. As she told me "I'm not someone who has ever articulated: I'm going to get married by the time I'm X and have Y number of children. It was probably something that I just took for granted—that that's just how many people's lives evolve...as you get older, you meet a partner and have a family. That just didn't seem to be happening for me."

"I found that as I was getting older, the number of new people I was meeting was becoming fewer and fewer. The work angle wasn't suitable for meeting anyone—there were males around, but not necessarily 'eligible' (although I know many people who met their partners through or at work)."

In a mad dash to beat the clock she too jumped on the internet and tapped away on dating sites hoping to land a forever man.

"I did the whole online thing. I blind-dated. I speed-dated. It went on and on. I made a few new male friends from it. I dated someone for a little while—he was commitment-phobic. But in the end, no 'success'. It did, however, provide great conversation fodder with my girlfriends—as we all seemed to be in a similar boat. We often shared and compared hilarious and horrendous online dating stories."

Along with the demise of her brief relationship, the thought of having children was pushed aside again as well as "it takes two to tango". When she was nearing forty she actively made the decision to have a family, but her options were now running out.

"Sometimes life doesn't work out the way you plan (or in my case, not plan). That's just the way it was. So I thought I needed to make a plan but in my case Plan A (or in other people's case, Plan B)."

Once Carmen had firmly planted the idea of going it solo, her now Plan A, she called her best friend to tell her. They both cried. Over the next four and a half years she relentlessly pursued becoming a mother. In fact, just after she passed her 39th birthday, she started on her first of seventeen fertility cycles.

The stakes were high; so was her anxiety. Her baby girl arrived after just a handful of cycles but with a wad of embryos stored she continued to do more rounds. She desperately wanted one more. "I wanted nothing more than my daughter to have a sibling. Someone else she could call her family, who'd be there for her, who was her blood. Unfortunately, that was never to be."

Carmen still refuses to calculate how much she spent over the years. At just under AU$10,000 a pop for a full stimulation round, which includes the doctor fees, medication, donor sperm components, hospital treatments and tests, it's pretty easy to gauge a ballpark figure. Some of this is covered by Medicare and there are some private health cover rebates available, but this amount doesn't include initial administration and donor program fees, embryos or sperm storage. Nor complementary therapies such as acupuncture or other 'herbal' treatments, travel costs for flights, accommodation and car hire when she was having to travel interstate for treatment and any other out of pocket expenses. She even had to sell her apartment in Melbourne to free up some finances.

Her situation was frustrating to say the least saying, "I do sometimes begrudge the fact that I have had to 'pay' to have a child whereas many people don't have to do that to have a family. Not that I begrudge my daughter. I have NEVER looked at her and thought about the cost. I would do it all again just for her. I no longer have that home as an asset, which means I have to start all over again – BUT I am debt-free. It's the price that I chose to pay in my endeavour to have my family."

"I'm just not sure if I want to acknowledge it because it doesn't change the outcome and what price can you put on having a child?"

My dear friend Georgie finally jumped into bed with Ivie Effe (IVF) after she gave up faffing about with a guy who wouldn't commit. She, like so many of us, got stuck in a relationship with a partner who agreed he wanted children, however, when push came to shove he was out the door. She ended their six-year relationship just after her 39th birthday. Only one month later, she began her solo motherhood journey, which had her use four different fertility clinics, to do six IUI rounds and two IVF cycles over five years of which she invested over sixty thousand US dollars.

She had success with the embryos created from her second round of IVF. Although she held off on the transfer of two of those embryos for two years due to work commitments, she finally implanted them when she turned 44. She told me "I was definitely giving it my last shot because I couldn't go through it all 'just one more time."

The fertility drugs had such an impact on Georgie mentally, physically and emotionally when things were not successful. She's now the very happy and exhausted mother of adorable twin girls. Oh and by the way, her ex is now in a relationship with a woman with 3 children!

Even though I considered us close friends, I hadn't connected with either girls in the flesh for many years due to the fact we were living different lives in different parts of the world. I knew Carmen had had a child through IVF thanks to social media, but I didn't know how to ask her about it. Same with Georgie; but it wasn't a conversation I felt I could casually ask about in messenger. It was probably through my own limited understandings of what using donor sperm meant for me at the time that I figured it was too awkward to ask them about it.

Early on, I mildly thought having a child solo was a sad thing to do. Not just emotionally sad but sad in the way that elderly ladies feel sorry for you. Like you weren't 'chosen' and you're one of the ones left on the shelf. I could imagine two old ducks having a good old frown down on how women are becoming mothers these days.

Esther: Oh, the poor lass can't secure or keep a husband.

Marge: I heard she had to go to a clinic to get pregnant.

Esther: What happens at a clinic?

Marge: Apparently, dear, they remove her eggs and put them in Petri dishes.

Esther: Oh!!! How do you make a baby out of a petri dish?

Marge: Oh you silly old chook. They add sperm.

Esther: Whose sperm is it?

Marge: I don't know. It's just how I've heard they do it these days.

Esther: Why don't they just do it how we did it... the old fashioned way?

Case in point. Child creation and family formation have evolved. For better or worse.

IVF was officially born in 1978 in England when baby Louise Brown successfully arrived. She was the first child to be welcomed into the world with the assistance of ART. Assisted Reproductive Technology was originally developed to assist couples, mainly women with blocked or missing fallopian tubes, who were having trouble conceiving. These days business is open to a much wider slew of people with all sorts of infertility issues.

I may have felt there were 'sad' connotations attached to choosing assisted reproductive technologies to create a much-desired family. My initial thoughts revealed so much about how out of touch, four billion dollars out of touch, I was with where the world was at with making babies.

I was also ignorant about the intricacies and nuances of creating baby miracles. I didn't know how hard it could be. I didn't know that there's really only a 24-hour window that women have for their best shot at falling pregnant. I didn't know how heavy the emotional burden was when trying to conceive. I didn't know it wasn't our birthright to create and produce a healthy baby. I didn't know any of this stuff until it affected me personally. I just didn't know.

Georgie and Carmen's stories also scared the bejesus out of me. All those punishing cycles. The drugs. The emotional torment. The money. On the flipside, I couldn't overlook the fact they were successful in their quests. They were both now mothers. They also helped break down my initial JUDGEMENT about this idea of being a solo mum and the process to become one. I saw them as strong, courageous women, but I still needed time to absorb my harsh reality. I wasn't sure I could emulate them or felt I needed to just yet. I guess in all honesty, I needed to experience the full gamut of emotions and absorb the sheer enormity of this plight.

For all the reasons that others may have difficulty in conceiving, mine like my two girlfriends was just due to the fact we were single.

At this juncture, all men were walking sperm to me. I studied their physical attributes weighing them up as assets or liabilities when combined with mine. Every man I came into contact with was sperm donor potential. The barman who served me three nights ago. Mister Barista. Even the guy with the big guns beating on his drum by the beach.

It was serendipitous that my good friend Pim had relocated to Australia not long after me. Miraculously, he bounced into the trendy seaside town of Byron Bay in NSW (New South Wales) just weeks after I had arrived. He, in his fine physical form, was the perfect upright sperm specimen. He was so close I could smell him. Recently single. Childfree; I saw this as a positive as maybe he would like to see how well his genes fared in the way of a little Johnny or Janie without giving up his gregarious lifestyle. He was stag-tastic, came from good stock and had a great life outlook. He was adventurous so would likely be up for it. He wouldn't fight me for custody or want to bring up a child (I don't think).

I only had to gather the courage to ask him. Oddly enough, I found it difficult to do. Instead, I tested the waters by joking with him on the phone about my baby plan. I told him that if he was up for it, he could be my backup genetic material, my Plan C as I already had a Plan B in place (well I was simultaneously working on one). He laughed along with me and said it had to be done the old-fashioned way. That was when the air came out of my idea. There was no way I could bring myself to get horizontal and roll around with my friend (yet). Mainly because I knew it could complicate things and potentially get very messy—emotionally and legally.

For some reason it unnerved me and seemed reckless. Still, it wasn't enough for me to completely wipe him as a back-up plan. If I'm really honest, I just wasn't ready to let go of finding my life mate. I felt I had to give finding LOVE one more go. So I did what any heartbroken single girl would do while sitting at home, I began online dating.

*Chapter 9*

# Seed Dating

*"Never date a woman you can hear ticking."*
*- Mark Patinkin, author*

*"Basically, dating is like climbing a volcano and you never
know when it's going to erupt, dumping molten lava and
burning you." - Robin Bielman, USA Today bestselling author*

DATING AT FORTY IS VERY different to dating at twenty or even thirty. The likelihood of meeting someone who has never been married, is without kids, is around the same age, wants a family, wants to get married, is fit and healthy, financially stable and cares about others beyond himself is rare. My friends convinced me to get into online dating before the puffiness around my eyes had subsided. That's the beauty of the internet, I didn't have to lay with tea bags over my eyes or enlist a makeup artist to put me together just so I could be seen in public. Nope. I didn't even have to get out of my pyjamas or slap on a spot of makeup to chat to a bunch of (maybe) single blokes.

Dating actually put a lot of pressure on me, but this was my new two-pronged approach. One, find a worthy 'for life' man; two, make a baby. I was outcome oriented, expecting a lot within a very tight timeframe, so the need for speed-to-seed was key. I was now in Brisbane for good, or at least while I figured the baby thing out, so jumped on the speediest dating apps there are—Tinder and Bumble—and began swiping away.

*"You gotta kiss some toads to land your prince."*
*- Kim, DSS Crusade Committee*

Of the few men I swiped right for, Patrick was one of them. I wasn't really drawn in by his photos but after deleting hundreds of profiles in minutes he was one of the few that had all his clothes on and actually included a paragraph of written text. He ran his own business and seemed to have his shit together. I felt he was worthy of a wave exchange.

He responded almost instantly and was quick to take our chat outside of the app that night and to a nearby bar. I arrived and ordered a drink before he got there and then sat wondering if I really cared to meet this person. I didn't have a whole lot to give emotionally, but I knew the prize was worth the effort. I was driven to secure a ring and some seeds. Not overnight, but before the year closed out.

An hour-long drink was all it took to secure a second date, which was a sweet midweek catch up soaking up the city skyline on a balmy January night. It was all very lovely but I couldn't be sure if Pat batted for the other team and he just didn't know it yet. Nevertheless, I scored a hattrick with Patrick as our conversation rolled over to date number three where he whisked me away on a two-hour drive south for a splash at a popular swimming spot back near the place I had only just left, Byron Bay.

To my surprise, it was a nudist tea tree lake located off the beaten track down an unsealed gravel road alongside a nudist beach. Not really knowing me, my mind swung into overload as I processed a thousand thoughts as to why he would bring me here. My smile concealed my perturbed frown and concern.

The sun's rays were laser strong and the watering hole was bathtub warm. Nudists basked around the edges soaking up the heat that dappled through the trees. Patrick stripped down to his tight Euro togs and jumped straight in. It took me a little longer to disrobe to my bikini and slide into the murky brown pond. The tannins from the tree leaves had stained the water turning it into a dark pool of grubby, brown liquid. I would normally be highly appreciative of the sentiment for bringing me to this highly spiritual piece of landscape that's revered for its healing powers, but this patriarch had really missed the mark. It looked anything but fresh, light and revitalising.

I wondered if that was the same for this date. I was still confused about Patrick's sexuality but decided to just go with his lead and maintain an open mind. The hours quickly passed as we chatted and frolicked about. He then held me close and scooped up handfuls of mud from the basin floor and trickled it all over my body, and all over my blue and white bikini which was now stained in two shades of turd. I didn't find this sexy; I found this, whatever this was, a little creepy.

Perhaps, that was because I couldn't get a read on Patrick's motives and there was no immediate spark between us, well, for me anyway. You can bet your bottom dollar that if I was there with Brad Pitt, I would be telling a completely different story. Something along the lines of, "He seduced me at a nudist lake by smearing revitalising mud all over my nearly naked body." There is no way I wouldn't find that hot as hell. But rolling about with Patrick in this poo brown sediment surrounded by nudies jiggling their pink bits like Lipton's Tea Bags was straight up weird and it really threw me.

I couldn't quite put my finger on why I felt this way but figured it was because I really wasn't that into him. It wasn't like I could call it for what it clearly was and go home. We were miles from there and it was a long walk to town. So I did what I always do——compensated by babbling on and dismissing my questionable thoughts.

Our conversation deepened over lunch which turned into afternoon cocktails. With a light head buzz, we tottered off to the beach for a quick sea clean before heading back to the pond for a final dunk and then home. It had been a long day and although I was confused by this man, I made the most of it. We caught the final shades of pink as they coloured the sky, which was a nice way to end out this weird day. Getting to know more about him over the course of the day, I asked him to share some of his craziest tales from when he lived in New York City. Once he started sharing, it's like his whole persona, and what was lurking below, finally made its way to the surface.

He revealed X rated stories of threesomes and orgies of days gone by. I nodded along listening, while at the same time, wondering why he was revealing this information to me. Was he digging for a reaction or just digging himself into a muddier hole? Or was he just playing me to get off on my reaction? He seemed to be super sexually adventurous and I couldn't imagine how one person, or one gender, could satisfy him long term.

His conversation took a disturbing twist when he shared a scenario about an ex-girlfriend. Apparently, she liked to be abused. So much so, she once asked him to take her out of town to a forest, tie her up, assault her and then leave her roped around a tree. He complied and then went shopping for three hours before returning to find her in an irate state. According to him, she raved about how much she loved the thrill of it all. From then onwards, they had to up the ante with something even more impassioned and abhorrent.

My frown returned to my face. The landscape setting for his last anecdote seemed to replicate the one we were in. As I listened, I questioned if this was his (perhaps watered down) side of the story. In which case, what was hers? Actually, it didn't matter. It seemed Patrick was very comfortable bringing me into his zone, however, I wasn't so comfortable being in it. I guessed he was either testing me or was clueless about dating.

Either way, it couldn't halt my eggs from quivering and wilting as he splashed about with the other shrivelled swimmers. I promptly patted 'Pat the Swamp Rat' goodbye and shook off the dirt he left on my mind, body and bikini.

I sailed straight into a date the following week with the slick Mr Yachty McSnobby. He ran his own boating business that took him around the world to play and ogle over rich boy toys. He arrived at the restaurant before I did and was waiting for me with wine in hand. He was friendly, classy and took total control of our date. These initial first twenty-five minutes scored him a big thumbs up. However, as the night wore on, his BF potential and shininess wore off.

He was on the hunt for a woman to merge into his world and fly around the planet together as a family with his two children. I, however, could only feel the pain of my wings being sawn off. A sensation I was all too familiar with. For some reason, I seemed to flit about with men who preferred to cage me in. Too scared to see me soar, I was only free to take flight like a kite attached to a string.

I didn't feel a connection with him and even though he offered a minuscule amount of hope for siring another lass, it would come at a huge price. Time. He said he would consider giving a new woman in his life the chance to be a mum down the track if he felt she would make a good one. Oh, really a test. Urgh! I've done enough dating training and tests over the past 25 years thanks. So Mr Yachty became a big, fat Mr Snobby Yachty McNotty. Cue Enya and sail away, sail away, sail away.

I had major physical chemistry with Tinder date number three. He instantly grabbed my curiosity when he revealed he brokered seeds for a living. Little did he know I was on a seed mission! He then clinched the attention of my loins when setting up our first dinner date when he inquired if I ate swimmers. Bam... I found my (seed)man! Our sassy banter lasted a week, which then rolled into a three date weekend.

We coasted along from that day forward for a few more weeks. The issue was, Seedman had legs but I promptly found out he had no tails. Well, to be fair he had tadpoles but his vas deferens, aka 'the kill-joy fishing net', blocked the chance of just one swimmer making a lucky break. Seedman's infertility was the final flag for me to kill flirting about and wasting time on Tinder dinners and get back to scrolling donor swimmers. The chances of me meeting that man who would be my life partner, the father or my children, my best friend, a man I'd marry, was about as probable as a drug-free IUI insemination—a sucky 4 per cent.

I had to accept that the chances of meeting 'the one' on Tinder, fall madly in love and be completely aligned at 41 years old when we've both accumulated a bunch of baggage was not an ideal route, especially, when the fertility window is tight.

I found myself cruising dating sites specifically with a baby making agenda and it was not ideal. Based on their image and words, I deciphered if they would be a good father. Did they really want kids as much as I did? Could I make it happen with them in less than twelve months? What would our lives look together as a family from the get-go? There were one or two at first glance that ticked all the same boxes as me, but just because we were perfect on paper that wouldn't make us a perfect couple, let alone perfect parents.

I wasn't nuts about seed-dating. It was seedy. So I finally traded it in for what I thought had better returns, the seed bank.

## Chapter 10

# Donor Swimmers over Tinder Dinners

*"Not without a shudder may the human hand reach into the mysterious urn of destiny." - Friedrich Schiller, poet*

*I HAD BEEN UMMING AND* ahhing about this ART path for so long because I really still hoped 'he' was out there. The little girl in me so wished I could just pull out an old but perfect Ken doll from the top shelf of a cupboard, dust him off and bring him back to life. He was the man I had grown up with my whole life, the one I was setting myself up for. Only he wasn't life sized and nothing about him was real life.

My mind really was still in a fog and my confidence in the pits following my relationship breakdown with Ian and those shitty dating experiences. And they weren't just shitty because in the flesh they didn't meet my expectations; they were shitty because they couldn't fit with my intention on my clock. Biology may be a non-negotiable, but it's become increasingly tweakable because of ART and I was thankful for its existence. I finally made an appointment with a fertility doctor.

At first, it was comparable to a therapy session with me divulging details and awkwardly explaining why I was there...alone. Like I was the first single woman ever to sit opposite him and tell him my sob story. Rather than be too open about being a spinster, I tried to spin some other story to throw him off my single scent. Something along the lines of "My boyfriend and I live in other parts of the world and we can't figure it out."

He didn't offer too much in the way of comfort before directing me to the bed next door for a transvaginal ultrasound.

On my back, pants down and covered with a white sheet, he then came in with gloves on, pulled the curtain across me and inserted the wand-like gadget up into my pelvis. He was a little wizard like so before we had a chance to create magic together, I dubbed him Doc Merlin. We both watched the screen intently as he waved it about. I couldn't see much other than some blurry shaped lines and even then I struggled to make something out of them. Magically two eggs appeared on the screen, one on each side. Both of which brought him much delight.

He removed the wand from my vagina, took off his gloves, told me to get dressed and meet him back in his office. There he delivered my diagnosis. "You're socially infertile!"

I didn't even know what that meant. I think I must have sat there confused for a moment while he told me I was good to move forward with treatment and that it was promising for me to have a baby before I was 42. With this news and my new socially infertile title, I paid my AU$570 and headed over to the nurse to take me through step by step the process of each treatment.

The IUI (Intrauterine insemination) is the least invasive method and the cheapest. It's often the first treatment women start with on their fertility journey. It involves having sperm placed through the neck of the cervix and into the uterus a day or two prior to ovulation using a speculum, syringe and catheter. With your legs spread and a nurse watching on, the doc opens the baby gateway with what seems like a giant clamp that could probably lift a small car for a tyre change.

Before the sperm worms are thrust up into the great unknown, the minuscule sample is washed to separate them from the semen in order to remove any substances such as chemicals and disease-carrying material, which are known cervix antagonisers that may provoke cervical hostility and adverse reactions. It's kind of like space invaders where your body defends itself from any foreign objects that infiltrate this territory.

Unfortunately, it's no time to play games, and you want your body to warmly welcome these visitors with open labia.

The sperm is also blended with a culture medium so the sperm will have something to 'swim in', which is then drawn up into a syringe. Armed with what hopefully is the liquid of life, the doc then inserts the catheter to the very top of the fallopian tubes and slowly empties the contents.

All in all, it takes about five to seven minutes from 'hello doc' to 'thanks and have a good afternoon'. Once he and the nurse leave, you can pull out your best attempts of an upside down ballerina pointe. Anything to possibly assist those tadpoles in finding their way.

Around the globe, IUI procedures aren't actually that successful overall. Less so at my age. If you're around the 40 years age mark, willing to inject yourself with hormone stimulating drugs, then there's about a 13 per cent chance one will hit the jackpot. Without, as I said above, just 4 per cent.

IVF, (In Vitro Fertilisation) on the other hand, does offer a little more hope, but it's a whole lot more intrusive requiring the daily stimulating injections and general anaesthesia to collect the eggs, a buddy to come and collect you after the harvest as well as a follow up visit for the implantation. For an old duck just as myself, there's about an 11 percent chance of success. The odds are much better for women under 35 who have around a 40 per cent chance of success.

I learned ICSI (Intracytoplasmic Sperm Injection) is probably the most specific ART procedure available, and its success is comparable to IVF. With ICSI, a single sperm is injected directly into the centre of an egg. Once the sperm and egg have hopefully connected, the embryo can then be transferred to the cervix the following day. At the time I went through the fertility clinic, it had approximately a 35 per cent pregnancy rate for women up to 35 years and 11 per cent for women who are 40 years of age.

My head was spinning fast with all the info she threw at me. Some of it stuck. Most did not. I was too busy trying to understand why I was infertile. I had never had any reproductive problems, Mrs Menses visited monthly and I was in good health.

The nurse had to almost click her fingers between my eyes to break me from my deep thought. I asked her how it was possible that I was infertile. She assured me I was physically fine (for now), but I was single, which, consequently at my age, pushed me into the socially infertile category.

Sheesh! It was a blow to my head, that's for sure. Another wake-up call, too. Not that I wasn't already feeling the urgency of my predicament, but speaking to specialists about such a personal topic only further heightened it. And I was certainly not alone. I found out that a high percentage of people turning to IVF are single women. In fact, more than half the people that walk through the same doors I did are solo flyers.

As a single woman, your 'why' for being there doesn't matter. You're instantly labelled as socially infertile. It was confronting to hear. It was also one of the rare times I had found myself in a minority group. While we both have the same sperm issue or lack thereof, same-sex women couples are at least in a relationship. I felt like I had been discarded by society and had just been moved from my huge poo pile and added to the reject heap.

Who decides this shit anyway? WHO that's who! The World Health Organisation (WHO) sets the benchmark for classifying infertility. It's officially defined by them as "the inability to conceive after one year of unprotected intercourse (six months if the woman is over age 35) or the inability to carry a pregnancy to live birth

Social Infertility is a term conceived by the Fertility industry directed at women who require donor sperm and fertility treatment to achieve pregnancy. For women hitting the middle-aged mark, this translates as 'you've left it too late!' It was a big, fat 'I'm Very Fucked' slap in the face.

Every time my ovulation came and went, I reflected upon it as a window of lost opportunity. It took me twenty-eight days to masterfully produce a voluptuous egg while waiting for Mr Tadpole to arrive. Once she, my egg, realised he, Mr Taddie was a 'no show', she would collapse in a flood of red rage.

I know fertility isn't a state of mind but there was no way I couldn't hold a pregnancy. I totally believed that. For me, it was because the arrows weren't being fired at the right time. Or ever. When the doctor quizzed me about my "partner", I entertained the idea of saying that there really was one on the scene but he just wasn't around right now.

My chat with Merlin took me straight back to the time when Ian booked us into a hotel for a week of decompression. I was ecstatic as I knew that his arrival was going to coincide with my ovulation window. In a wide-eyed single, white, frenzied female kind of way, I saw this as an open opportunity to take advantage of this situation by "shoplifting the pootie" as Rod Tidwell explains to Jerry Maguire he's done in the movie,

Jerry Maguire. In my instance, though, I wasn't pilfering the pootie...just the materials required to create one.

I had six nights to achieve this mission and even though a doona dance can be the key to a fast connection, ours was still operating at dial-up speed. He was exhausted from work. While I managed to secure a few successful climbs of his erect fort, I could have done with a physical set of defibrillator paddles to give the spark between us some actual spark.

Unbeknown to him, I had finally put my long-held suppressed desire to be a mother front and centre. I secretly started having fertility acupuncture in a bid to keep my eggs well-nourished in my incubator while I figured out our baby strategy over the next year or so. I'd been stoking and reviving them with needles and Chinese herbs as well as oxygenating stagnant blood with cupping therapy.

I had also just completed a week-long Vedic Meditation course to not only keep me closer to the tracks when I was unravelling but also to silence my inner voices at any time throughout my nutso baby-making exploration.

While I was sad he got back on that plane and headed north without me, I was left with hope that perhaps he had left something behind in me. The next ten days were horrendously long. Daylight savings didn't help with drawing out the days either. I became obsessed with Googling every little change or symptom in my body that could pertain to pregnancy and was thrilled to find evidence supporting my every beguiled thought.

When my period never showed up two weeks later nor the following month, I delved deeper into the web's online forums to confirm I was indeed up the duff. Incredibly sore boobs? Yes. Peeing in the middle of the night? Yes. A headache? Yes. Spotting day before my first period and a skipped second one? Yes. Pink and brown spotting when I wipe? Yes.Oh my, according to all the forum advisors on selected posts, I was pregnant.

The following day I went to a chemist and purchased a couple of home pregnancy kits. The sales assistant asked me if this was the first time I was doing a test. I responded, "Yes, but I KNOW I am pregnant." As she ran my sale, she said, "Congratulations." I walked away wrapped up in a smug (aka shrug).

That confidence soon faded and turned into confusion once my pee on the stick worked its magic. Or in this case, it's failed magic. It came back with a BFN. A BIG FAT NEGATIVE! I didn't believe the result and decided I'd wait a day or two to do another test.

Of course, it too came back negative. I then decided that the pregnancy tests failed and the truth would be revealed through a blood test.

I went to a local medical centre and told the doctor I thought I was pregnant and had done two home tests, but that they were wrong. He didn't seem too impressed having to send me off just to have his suspicions confirmed through a blood test but did so anyway. Three days later I went back to see him and get my result. Again, it was a BFN. I was still convinced I was pregnant and the blood tests were wrong. None of this made sense. After all, I still hadn't had my period in over two months.

I called Kim, who at the time worked in a pharmacy, and told her how I hadn't had my period. She was quick to say it was highly likely to be a 'phantom pregnancy', something I dismissed while her words ricocheted out of my phone. But it was enough to stir me and set me off on a Google search to learn more.

The headline of the first article I brought up in bold type read, "Your mind is pregnant not your body." Ah, shit balls. This really was a thing. I read on.

"A phantom pregnancy, also known as ghost pregnancy is when the woman's mind convinces her body that a baby is present." It went on to say something like "these pregnancies mimic real ones and may have some or all of the classic symptoms of pregnancy such as morning sickness, the absence of menstruation, swollen breasts, nipple changes, lactation and even an enlarged abdomen."

I could feel myself sinking further down my bed under my doona. "Its medical term is Pseudocyesis. It most commonly emerges in women who are desperate to conceive and long for a baby." Gulp. "And they convince themselves and others that they are indeed pregnant."

But it's not like they just make it all up. There are actual body changes that take place because a woman's endocrine system and pituitary gland are influenced to secrete pregnancy specific hormones–specifically oestrogen and prolactin. Secreted prolactin does play a role in enlarging the breasts and preparing them for lactation.

Women with pseudocyesis can even throw health professionals as they can be so convincing that they are also fooled into thinking the ladies are pregnant!

I was shocked to read that some women even believe they are pregnant right up until they go into (false) labour. It's only at this point that their pregnancy does a Trey-The-Ghoster on them.

This was another one of those moments when I realised that I wanted a baby so badly I couldn't shove the idea back in the box. So much so, I even wished my period away. It wasn't until month three that the red floodgates opened, and I cried me a river. I had made my mind up that this was my opportunity to land a baby but energetically my body said no. This time my gut wasn't sending me mixed messages, it was my mind. I had been ghosted on again.

Even though there wasn't a lost baby to mourn, there was still a loss. I had lost hope.

Reluctantly, Ian agreed to try a couple of times for a baby. But his efforts were half-arsed as he did not want to bend to my demanding biological timeframe. While he was less than enthusiastic in assisting me in fighting for my cause, to his credit, he did throw me a few swimmers but they didn't 'come' freely.

I persuaded him to have his semen, urine and blood tested to find out if he would even medically qualify to be a baby dadda. He was a social drinker and had at times been a packet a day stress smoker. Surprisingly, a week later his results came back as 'pretty good', but not surprisingly, we most definitely were not.

This was not the way he or I wanted to create a child. A child deserves better. I knew that. In my mind though, Ian was my only and last hope. I was prepared to do whatever it took to squeeze any semen out of him. At one point I even tried to sell him on the idea that he could be the donor of my child. He could finally be a father, I told him, and I'd ask for nothing of him.

That's what's so insane about the vociferous ticking of the biological clock. If women choose to tune into it. Not all of us do but once you hear it, and march to its tempo, it has the capacity to send you more cuckoo than a cuckoo clock can.

And Adam knows this all too well. He's the guy who has been managing the Sperm Donation Australia (SDA) Facebook page for nearly five years. He shared some pregnancy stories with me and boy does he have some rippers with one in particular that stood out.

He told me that one woman got really desperate when she couldn't get a donor for one insemination cycle so she jumped on Tinder to fill the gap. Unfortunately for her, her date wouldn't have a one night stand without using a condom. As he said, "No glove, no love."

She conceded and once their romp was over, she promptly kicked him out then fished the used rubber out of the trash, turned it inside out and inserted it into her uterus.

No. It didn't work.

Ian had me on top and upside down in both hemispheres. Clearly, we weren't successful in our epic global jiggy jaunts. We only ever had unprotected sex when we hooked up, and I'd rarely ingested a contraceptive pill in my life. I wasn't asked if we used any kind of natural contraceptive measures such as withdrawal, avoided sexual activity during the fertile window or if we even did the doona dance at all.

It was irrelevant because I was there in the clinic on my own.

Noticeably, I was single. Even if I was still hopeful of a miraculous reconciliation.

The doc picked up what I was putting down. And now I was branded as socially infertile. A label fitted me like a leather mini skirt. It not only didn't fit, it ethically rubbed me the wrong way and it was ridiculous. What a social shift slap!

Before I could move forward with any treatment at the clinic, I had to get a bunch of tests done. These included general bloods, STIs (Sexually Transmitted Infections) and a top up vaccination for chickenpox.

While the vaccination for chickenpox was not mandatory, the implications for me not having it far outweighed the risk.

Had I not seen firsthand the result of a friend's baby who contracted the disease inside her womb, I may not have bothered. This child was unfortunately born with major physical defects. Despite now leading a relatively normal life, her 'normal' includes regular hospital visits and continual operations.

Once my tests came back a few days later AOK, I was given the green light to go on a sperm spree in the sperm store. This was an Ahhhhhh moment. I finally felt as though I was making headway and there really, truly was a way for me to be a mother on my own.

Once I had access to the sperm store, aka donor library, my prime dating nights were then spent perusing potential donor profiles, expanding their pictures into large, fuzzy blobs on my computer screen, and going over genetic details with a fine tooth comb.

'Donor Deciding' was vastly different to 'Seed Dating' as nailing down some seeds was a sure thing. It may have meant picking up the bill at the end of the night, and a very expensive one at that.

When I had access to the clinic's "spank bank", local donor semen specimens were AU$240 each for half a millilitre vial and AU$1270 for an imported one with the same volume. There were so few Aussie natives to choose from, so it was highly likely my potential baby would have international roots.

Controlling how the night went down and who I ended up with was satisfying. This was so much better than Tinder. Rather than go on dates with men and scrutinize their physical attributes and entertain pointless conversation, I could save myself the time and discomfort of squeezing into my little black dress, or as we women refer to it as the LBD, by hanging at home scrolling through legitimate baby making potentials.

Yes, I avoided the pain of sitting through a bunch of excruciating dates and any motherhood scrutiny that came my way; like that of my failed night out with Mr Yachty McSnotty.

I could also dally about with different species of man. One cycle I could choose a tall, athletic blonde. The next, give a computer brainiac a whirl. I could do this with one straightforward, smooth, fast transaction while in the comfort of my activewear while curled up on the couch.

At the time, this 'ugly-dip' as some women refer to it, offered far more hope than dating. Securing seed was a sure thing. So, instead of finding 'The One' to create my child with, I decided I would manufacture that special one myself. Of course, if another special 'one' came along with his own set of favourable digits, such as a 40-odd-year-old, well-built 6 foot something, well then that too would be more than OK.

Counselling was mandatory for me when I was pursuing IUIs through the fertility clinic. It expanded my awareness and allowed me to get outside my head about what solo parenting looked like for me once a baby made its way into the world. I think we think we know, but it's not until it's a conversation beyond the one you have with your internal guiding forces that you gain a much larger perspective. The potential issues and concerns that were discussed in my counselling session were not exclusively tied to the outcome of using an anonymous donor either.

I met with the psych who talked me through scenarios so I could better get a grasp on what going through with IVF meant. When you're completely consumed with "I want a baby" desires or perhaps more flippantly believe "giving sperm is just like giving blood", you're not necessarily deeply aware of the little matters that may pop up or the long term ramifications of your actions, thoughts and/ or desires you have today.

She reiterated that a child born with the assistance of IVF using donor sperm would not have access to the father until they were 18 years old. In some places though, the age may be sixteen years old. I was probed about how I'd respond to the myriad of questions from my child, how I would cope as a single mother, as well as the emotional roller coaster of the IVF process and ensuring I had a support system in place.

IVF clinics want to ensure that you fully understand that there could be multiple children birthed around the globe from the same sperm donor, and your potential child or children, could have a bunch of siblings. They want to know your thoughts about how you think you'd feel if you received a random call out of the blue saying, "I'm related to your child and I'd love to meet them."

It was in the session with the psych that I learned that if I had a bunch of viable embryos left over and I had one, or a few successful births, then I could not donate them. I could only keep them for myself for as long as I could keep paying for the freezing fees or my other option was to destroy them. They do this because the donor will not have agreed to a second party having access to and using their sperm.

Let's just say, all this new information was just a tad overwhelming and seemed like a bigger responsibility than I had wanted for myself. It was potentially a byproduct of combining donor conception with ART though.

I was curious about how I would go about using my friend Plan C Pim as my donor and what the implications of that might be.

The counsellor discouraged the use of known donor semen as she felt it would put me at risk legally in regards to child care payments as well as co-parenting struggles. She told me that the contracts outside a clinic don't stand up legally in court and parental rights can get muddy. Each parent can have opposing thoughts about what level of involvement they are qualified for, and it can be an ever-changing argument as the child grows.

One implication that I was unaware of was how the donor's parents might feel if I were to have a child; that is that they had a grandchild that they would never get to see or perhaps even know about. Pim had no children of his own and so his parents would not be regarded as my child's grandparents. I realised this could be quite hurtful and heartbreaking for them. A total quagmire.

Our conversation definitely gave me some things to think about as I drove home.

Until I was in this position pursuing motherhood, I would never have known that infertility was so prolific. I really did believe it was every woman's right if she chose it, and something I never had to worry about; of course, until I did. I was shocked to learn that around 12 per cent of women in the USA have received infertility services in their lifetime. *(2006-2010 National Survey of Family Growth, CDC).*

Research done by the University of NSW in Sydney revealed these horrible 2015 stats: Of the 77,721 initiated ART cycles, 63,848 (82.2 percent) resulted in either an embryo transfer or all oocytes/embryos being cryopreserved. Of the initiated cycles, 22.8 per cent (17,726) resulted in a clinical pregnancy and 18.1 per cent (14,040) in a live delivery.

You can understand why assisted reproductive services have made such an impact globally and are a multi-billion dollar money-making business. I chose the career path over having a family and therefore, plain and simple, it was my fault. I could be classified as selfish for having a career and remaining child-free but can also be called the same for pursuing solo-motherhood. These days, though, it didn't make sense that I couldn't have both.

While I've spent a good chunk of time reflecting over the infertile label, not one of my relationships in the past ten years had the staying power to get me, or us, to child creation. I tried. But it wasn't to be. I even fought for and justified the wrong relationship just to get me across the motherhood line.

Ten months after my first fertility clinic appointment, I finally decided it was time to start moving forward with an IUI procedure. I had delayed it for so many months as they were a last-ditch effort of keeping the doors open for meeting someone. I had so hoped I'd have met 'the one' by now or Ian would have randomly woken up realising what a mistake he had made letting me go. Neither was to be.

It also took me all this time to come to grips with moving forward with this alone and to be honest, I still had to shake off my own judgements I had about myself needing to go down this avenue. I hadn't really been that tuned-in to notice the full impact JUDGEMENT had on me. It too was along for the ride and every now and then, unconsciously, it had been dispensing directions from the boot of the car.

I had been carrying some other negative thoughts along with tons of SHAME about this whole journey. All of it. My past choices. My present predicament. My future choices. The realisation that no one wanted to marry me. That I still wasn't worthy of being proposed to. That I was that reject, who had to do this alone.

Thankfully, a light flickered in one tiny dark corner of my body, where I had stored a little belief that I was quite a catch for someone out there. So, it wasn't all bleak. But I really, really did want someone to hold my hand. Share a child with. A wingman to be by my side until he or I died.

Time, however, had run out.

I turned the volume down on my internal dialogue then picked up the phone and called the clinic nurse. This was the beginning of living my life dictated by ovulation (ovu) cycles.

Despite holidaying in Townsville for a chunk of the summer, we still coordinated an IUI procedure within the week. I felt this was the least invasive method and I wanted to move forward drug-free. She emailed me some forms so I could get blood tests done at a nearby local pathology to gauge my hormone levels, which change when the egg has been released.

Luteinising hormone (LH) spikes giving a clear indication that it's prime injecting slime time. I also had an internal scan by a local fertility doctor to see if there was an egg waiting on my follicle. I was stoked to discover there were two bubbles of potential joy (18mm and 20mm) waiting to be kissed on my left ovary.

I then waited to hear from the doctor if we were on or not. Hours later I got the go-ahead for the next day. I then injected myself with a trigger shot of hormone human chorionic gonadotropin (hCG) just below my belly, which helps follicles mature and ensures that ovulation occurs within 36 hours. As an egg survives for only 12 to 24 hours post-ovulation, while sperm can live in the fallopian tubes for days, my appointment with the doc was set for 18 hours later.

The next morning, I jumped on a plane and headed to the sunny Gold Coast. While in transit, my wizard-like doctor evolved into becoming my fantasy beachside Latin lover. He had to. It was the only way I could process what I was doing. Yes, I was bringing some sexy to my IUI…

Once I landed, I raced over to the hotel room he had booked for us Here, he'd scattered crimson rose petals all over the crisp white floor tile and on the white satin sheets that sparkled like diamonds on the freshly made bed. The curtains swayed slowly as the warm, salty, sea breeze wafted through the window on this balmy afternoon. I barely had a moment to breathe it all in before his head was between my legs.

Very softly, he told me to relax and then propped me up a little, then… he inserted a clamp.

In that very instant, and with that ripping sound effect as loud as a thundercloud above, my charming Latin lover vanished, and I was left face taut and legs spread for you guessed it, Merlin, my 60 odd-year-old fertility doctor.

While I was shocked back to reality, at least he was armed with the sperm of a sexy, tall, dark-haired, green-eyed, 26-year-old Hungarian hottie, that was about to be squirted deep inside my cervix.

In reality, my IUI was a very stony experience, not a steamy one. There was no red hot-blooded lover and my sexy Hunk-arian's defrosted semen specimen arrived in a small clear canister. Sadly, it was no Tiffany box but I was hopeful there was one diamond in there. The cleaned semen sample had already had its useless junk removed and had been combined with half a mil of culture medium which was the same quantity as the sperm contents. The Hunk-arian was now known as code #3210. He was nameless, faceless and voiceless.

I lay semi-naked on a hospital bed with a sheet covering my nether regions waiting for the Doc's grand entrance. He cross-checked the canister's details on both the consent form and specimen label before signing off on it and then making his next moves to do the deed with me.

He drew #3-2-1-g0 up into the syringe then clamped my vagina with a speculum just as they do for pap smears. Then, with a catheter attached to a syringe, he inserted the semen to the top of my left fallopian tube where the two eggs waited for Mr Tadpole's arrival.

Our emotionless liaison lasted all of seven minutes. Then, Doc Merlin vanished and I was left with my legs in the air squeezing my vagina tight. I did an entire year's worth of Kegels hoping not a drop would dribble out.

Once I put myself back together, I paid the receptionist for my precious speck of fluid, drove to the airport and got on a plane out of there.

*"It is a well-documented fact that guys will not ask for directions. This is a biological thing. This is why it takes several million sperm cells to locate a female egg, despite the fact that the egg is, relative to them, the size of Wisconsin."*
*- Dave Barry, New York Times best-selling author.*

## 2WW (The Two Week Wait)

These next fourteen days, or three hundred and thirty-six hours, were painfully slow. I was in the gorgeous Queensland tropics enjoying this festive time of year with my mum, so I didn't mind that these relaxing weeks were drawn out. I relished the quiet, long, humid days that consisted of beach walks, lazy lunches, pool time and bingeing on movies.

This time, I stayed off the internet forums; didn't do extra pregnancy tests or Google every twitch, pain and movement; and tried to stay outside of my head. I was quietly confident that this year I was going to be a mother of a mini Magyar (Hungarian).

I was supposed to have a blood test on day twelve to see if the procedure was a success. In full holiday mode and self-assured, I didn't bother following up. Two days later that assurance was blown out of the water when Mrs Menses, aka Aunty Flo, showed up uninvited. My confidence took a direct hit; uncertainty and confusion then gained momentum.

JUDGEMENT had an opinion on the matter, too. Maybe I'm not an ideal host? I had been emotionally winded. The realisation that this was going to suck up some finances finally struck. Perhaps throwing down dollars was the test to see how much I really wanted this. What's it worth to me? Hmmm, perplexing thoughts.

Uncertain and disheartened, I pressed ahead with another two IUI cycles. Once more with the 'Hunk-arian' and another with a tall, dark-haired 28 year-old American chiropractor. Depressingly, neither worked.

Merlin was no medical magician and I was now deemed 'medically infertile.' I took to the mirror to observe my pain. As I looked deep into my eyes through the mirror's reflection, I could see defeat staring back at me. I started to unravel once again.

I knew my only option was to pull out the IVF big guns and harvest my eggs. I had foolishly passed the doctor-given expiration date for freezing my potential joy bubbles, and now I had no choice. This option, seemingly my only one, seemed ludicrous to me. I cried. A lot. It wasn't supposed to be this hard. It didn't make sense. Nothing in my life did.

Instead of immediately signing up for IVF for my forthcoming cycle, I somehow managed to reason with myself to put my spinning head, broken heart, bruised ego and deteriorating eggs in the fridge for a couple of months for a cooling off period. It was time to recalibrate and take a moment to breathe and reflect. I got small. I got quiet. It was in this space, I could faintly hear a whisper. As I tapped into it, the words became louder and clearer. Theories about my failed IUI's were surfacing.

"I'm old and my eggs are cooked," next it pivoted to, "Perhaps the doctor didn't execute at the right time?" and then the volume turned it up on, "The sperm is no good!" Whoa, now there's a thought! It was a light bulb moment that set me off to hold a microscope up over this topic by doing a stack of research, which revealed some surprising information, and inevitably, inspired me to write this book.

*Chapter 11*

# Girl Gone Rogue

*"You have the Answer. Just get quiet enough to hear it."*
*- Pat Obuchowski, author*

TIMEOUT. MENTAL BREAKS. VACATIONS. THEY'RE just what the doctor ordered, even though I didn't get a script for one. I took the liberty of doing that for myself by prescribing me some 'me time'. Once I lamented the losses of not falling pregnant and took a moment to sit still with my thoughts, I found a deeper strength to continue pressing ahead.

I was adamant that I wanted to create a baby but didn't feel IVF was right for me. Not yet anyway. I may have been delusional, but I didn't believe I was medically infertile. Nor did my DSS Crusade Committee.

This time, I would carve out my own way forward. I didn't exactly know how it would roll out, but I wasn't going to let that stop me.

I took stock of my pregnancy attempts thus far:
- Get back with a former boyfriend. Tried. Failed.
- Have ex-boyfriend be a donor daddy. Tried. Failed.
- Seed Dating. Tried. Failed.
- IUIs x 3. Tried. Failed.
- Make a baby with friend Pim. Plan C.
- ONS (One Night Stand). Nope. Can't do it.

I felt there had to be a solution out there and it was time to get really creative in order to find a realistic one. Adopting a baby was one, but as a single woman that had only just relocated back to Oz, I felt there were too many variables and the stakes too high. Besides, if Deborra-Lee Furness and Hugh Jackman couldn't even make it happen in Australia, what chance did I have? Zip! It's why Deborra created the organisation Hopeland, to better connect children with homes and families.

Three girlfriends offered me their eggs and another her womb, which was wonderful but these were not what I needed. Interestingly, none of these women offered me their partners taddies—and I was desperate for sperm not eggs or incubators. Clearly it was too close for comfort for them. I didn't mind. However, an intro to their hubby's brother or best friend would have been a nice offering!

So I threw myself at Dr Google for ideas and alternatives then actively started fleshing out a plan.

I took three approaches:
- A health and wellness one.
- A medical one.
- A research one.

Over the next three months, I sat at my local library for hours researching, reading and setting up appointments.

While I did that, I also contacted Doc Merlin to obtain a prescription for some backup drugs (Clomid) which helps initiate ovulation and a referral for a HyCosy procedure with a radiologist to rule out any obstructions in my uterus.

The radiologist I booked in with agreed with the doc which was encouraging. She said together they were a complementary pair and give me a really good chance.

A hysterosalpingogram (HSG) is an old-fashioned medical X-ray test that looks at the inside of the uterus and fallopian tubes once your insides have been squirted with water and an iodine-based dye. Sometimes the water soluble solution alone will help flush out any swimmer hurdles, but they're more often removed with a dose of poppy seed oil.

HyCoSy, shortened from Hysterosalpingo-contrast-sonography because it is just too goddamn hard to pronounce, is a newer techy ultrasound to check if your bits are out of sorts blocking your chances of falling pregnant. It's supposed to be less painful than an HSG, but that's just code for saying it's a little more exxy (expensive). There's also a HyFoSy, which you guessed it, not only rivals the HyCoSy with its uber long name, hysterosalpingo-foam sonography, it's a lot fancier than the other procedures as it uses foam to help mow down any obstructions.

Every time I see this word, my mind throws back to those popular foam parties of the nineties. Tearing up the dance floor to MC Hammer in a club with thick foam pouring out of hoses over sweaty bodies. Those were the days, and that foam often wiped the dance floor clear too.

If the soldiers still can't tunnel their way through, more invasive investigating can include a diagnostic laparoscopy or keyhole surgery, to examine what's going on inside the abdomen. This is more of a last resort when other tests haven't been able to provide enough information or insight for a diagnosis.

Next on my hit list was my GP again to request a general blood and STI test—to ensure Seedman hadn't planted any cooties, and to check to see if I still had any viable eggs. I also made an appointment at a prenatal care clinic at a nearby hospital. I did this as I wanted their opinion and to add more members to my cheering squad for further encouragement of my plight. I hoped they might have had other tests that could help get to the root cause of my "infertility". At the very least, I wanted some insight about my situation and some more moral support to confirm I wasn't fucking crazy!

Once I received the results from my GP, I had the confidence to continue soldiering on myself.

I went in for an AMH (Anti-Mullerian Hormone) check, which is a simple blood test that gives a good indication of how many eggs a woman has left by measuring the amount of hormone in her bloodstream. It also gives a quantitative guide to assess a woman's ovarian "age" but it doesn't inform you about egg quality. Nor does it tell you if you have complications such as endometriosis.

My AMH score had dropped a little (from 28 pmol/L to 21.9 pmol/L or 3.066ng/mL), which was expected, but I was still in the running for a bub. This was a vital step in me forging ahead and not stressing about missed ovulation cycles as much. I knew that by continuing to look after myself, I was only elevating my health and therefore creating better, healthier quality eggs. Had my AMH test result not come back so good,

I probably would have reconsidered turning to IVF as it would have been the swifter route.

Next, I needed to understand my reproductive system more deeply so I could be sure I knew exactly how my cycle worked. It had been a wee-while since I'd learned anything about reproduction. If I took a stab at it, I would have officially been ten years old and in grade six when I first got my 'these are girl's bits' and 'these are boy's bits' chat.

During class time we watched videos that were extremely awkward. If I recall, there was always one kid making silly jokes in the class while 32 sets of eyes blushingly watched a terribly produced documentary about what was happening to our bodies. Unofficially, my sex-ed began years before, playing show and tell with the boys who lived on my street.

I not only think it's really important to know how your body functions, but also have the capacity to really tune into what's going on. Both are imperative when trying to conceive.

For the sake of not complicating things, I'll only refer to my 28-day cycle. In an ideal woman's world, she too would have one of the average menstrual cycles, which lasts approximately four weeks. Day one of the cycle is the first day of a woman's period. Known also as menstruation, it's a result of the shedding of the endometrium, a mucous layer, which has grown in preparation for pregnancy during the previous cycle.

A lack of the right levels of hormones triggers this process to occur as it indicates to the body that no pregnancy is present. Two other hormones that are vital in the process of preparing the body for pregnancy and are released by the pituitary gland are FSH (follicle stimulating hormone) and LH (luteinising hormone). Together, they stimulate the ovary and cause follicle growth. As the follicle grows and develops it begins to secrete estrogen during the middle of a woman's cycle. This stimulates an LH surge, which results in the follicle rupturing and releasing the egg.

At this time, the fimbria of the fallopian tube sweep over the ovary and wave the egg into the tube. Meanwhile, the follicle that produced the egg produces progesterone to prepare the uterus with the rich endometrial lining needed for implantation; and ultimately to sustain pregnancy.

If intercourse has occurred, or sperm has been artificially implanted into the cervix, conception may occur. If so, then the fertilised egg travels through the fallopian tube toward the uterus where it will implant itself into the thick endometrial lining. This occurs on about Day 20 of the cycle.

The best possible chance to fall pregnant is on day 14 of a 28 day cycle. It can be on either side of that depending on your actual cycle length, which makes it tricky to pinpoint it to begin with.

Cervical hostility can be a major impediment for conception, too, and it's why IUIs potentially have a better chance of success.

As I touched on earlier, there are a lot of things within the woman's body that may be unfriendly to male sperm, including cervical mucus.

It's intended by nature to work as a guide, helping push sperm along through the vagina and into the cervix and beyond, as well as offer important nutrients to give the sperm the energy it needs for the long journey ahead. Unfortunately though, it can actually work against the sperm it's supposed to be assisting. Suiting up for battle, Ms. C Mewcus (cervical mucus) can actually go on the attack, killing sperm before they ever have a chance to make it to the awaiting egg.

Things like infection in the lower reproductive tract can cause the vaginal fluids to become tainted which can kill or damage sperm as they enter the vajayjay. Anti-sperm antibodies actually immobilize sperm, before they can even enter the cervix. IUI's are a way to avoid this conflict.

Mucus that helps sperm get into the womb has a raw egg white consistency. It's clear and wet and can be stretched between your fingers.

The mucus that is drier, white or hits your knickers in a glutinous chunk shows up outside of the fertile window. It's highly hostile and will shoot down soldiers that have been deployed to get through the womb.

The ideal picnic zone, as I call it, is one where it's a light breezy, blue sky, sunny day, with a few other groups of people around, but the park is not overcrowded, nor is it isolated. This picture is the perfect egg and sperm 'thrive n jive' alkaline environment.

A diet high in fruits and vegetables, as well as a healthy dousing of H2O, helps to keep the body in more favourable picnic conditions. Meats, processed foods, dairy and sodas tend to cause the body to become more acidic.

As a long time vegetarian, health coach and a 'raw' abiding citizen, known for my love of kale, I know my lifestyle choices have extended my egg shelf life. I took it up a notch by not consuming any gluten, caffeine, processed foods and sugar or dairy at all for six months.

While I steer clear of toxic chemicals in cleaning products, personal products, and fruits and vegetables as much as I can, it's not easy to get them out of your life completely. Especially with the way we live today. Many of these chemicals actually disrupt the body's endocrine system, the place where hormones are measured and dished out.

As discussed in chapter 7, our endocrine systems are made up of a number of hormones and related glands, including our ovaries. In a healthy environment they all work together to keep the reproductive system beautifully balanced.

When endocrine disruptors invade the body, though, they wreak havoc on hormones by mimicking and altering their levels. Endocrine disruptors creep into our lives in a number of ways. To avoid them you need to avoid these items:

- Chemical cleaning products including laundry and dishwashing detergents
- Personal care products such as cosmetics, shampoo, conditioner, soaps - anything with added fragrances
- Pesticides
- Plastic food containers and plastic bottles and avoid plastic wrapping to microwave food. This makes takeout food a nightmare!
- Other PVC (polyvinyl chloride or vinyl) infused products such as shower curtains and floor coverings
- Linings of metal food cans
- Baby and children's toys
- Decorative treatment products such as paints and varnishes
- Fatty animal products

This was a really important juncture for me because the process up until now had been very corporate clinical. To take matters into my own hands, I needed to ensure I was in great health to do so. My diet was, and always is in pretty good shape, so I opened my self-evaluation up even further then made an appointment to see a dentist. This may seem a little l left field. I mean, I want to get pregnant so what does perfect pearly whites have to do with it? Turns out a lot!

Gum disease or periodontal disease is a chronic, infectious and inflammatory disease of the gums and supporting tissues. Just like cavities, it's caused by plaque, which is a build-up of bacteria.

It's a naturally occurring thing that happens in every mouth which is why cleaning twice a day and flossing is important to remove it. It affects fertility due to the bacteria passing into our circulatory systems where it is then spread all around the body causing chronic inflammation. Apparently, according to studies I read, there's a link between periodontal disease and both endometriosis and polycystic ovarian syndrome too.

As I hadn't been in town long, I had to search my new local hood for a respected practice. I came across one that had a stack of five star reviews and was only five minutes from where I was. I called and made an appointment. Two days later, I arrived on their clinic doorstep only to be greeted by a Stepford Wife in a crisp pale blue shirt and navy pants.

I was chauffeured through to meet with another lady sitting at a desk behind a glass wall. She shook my hand and introduced herself while gesturing for me to sit down across from her. She then gave me the rundown of their processes before I was handed over to another Stepford wife who walked me down a corridor to finally meet the dentist, Rachelle. She also shook my hand and gestured for me to take a seat. I backed up into the only available seat, the dentist's chair. After fifteen minutes of meddling about in my mouth, instructing her assistant to take notes, Rachelle gave me her analysis. My pearly whites were in good shape but I had some gum inflammation.

I was flung across to another room to receive the dentist's findings and more investigating by another Stepford wife. Here, a young, preppy 20-odd-year-old was waiting to give me some deep gum cleaning and unsolicited therapy. With a sharp instrument between my teeth, essentially gagging me from responding, she began counselling me about the importance of health and finding balance in my life.

She obviously was unaware that my nickname was Kaley (which is why I called my health coaching business The Kaleo Way) and that I was on a desperate mission to secure sperm—two things I couldn't be bothered explaining. So I channelled my spirit animal, the dragon, took a deep breath to capture all those gurgling stomach gases and exhaled directly into her face. At the very least in my mind it had some effect, she was none the wiser with her face hidden behind her mask and glasses.

Inflammation shows up in various ways in the body, therefore, my inflamed thoughts also led me to a neuro therapist, for a type of biofeedback that uses real-time displays of electroencephalography (EEG) to change and improve brain functioning. I did this to help me refrain from looking backwards and beating myself up for the situation I was in.

I needed to get off my life loop, alter my usage of language, keep JUDGEMENT at bay and bolster my confidence in moving forward rogue style. After just a few sessions, my brain had been so jumbled and cleaned out that I could barely relate to the broken woman I was just six months prior.

It wasn't until I connected next with an 80 odd year-old medical scientist and professor, that I truly felt what I was doing was on track and OKAY! Receiving permission by the professor to seek out semen in an unconventional way gave me the 100 per cent encouragement boost I needed. I thought I had already given myself the go ahead, but it was his reassurance that made it very real for me to truly believe it was possible for me to be a mum.

My experience at the fertility clinic put me off kilter, took away the pep in my step, and pulled the rug from under my feet—all of it. That experience knocked me and even though I didn't believe the results were indicative of me and my situation, that shit did trickle into my psyche.

Both the neuro-therapist and my gal pal Kim had independently told me about Professor Cliff Hawkins, and his work with fertility, which led me to phoning him and sharing my story. I was blown away that he actually was available to take my call.

I informed him of my infertile classification. He immediately balked. I then told him the short PG version of my baby-making journey so far. He was quick to encourage me to immediately send all my recent blood work results over to him so he could assess them. He responded within 24 hours to reassure me that I was a perfectly healthy 41-year-old woman who he didn't believe was infertile. He predicted that my fertility issue wasn't with me physically, but that the real issue was that I lacked access to fresh, quality sperm.

It's amazing that once you feel that someone gets you, it allows all that crazy to just melt away. It was a break-through conversation for me and a huge turning point as his words gave me the confidence to keep pressing forward outside IVF. It was like he had just given me the big AOK that I needed.

Among his research, he really focused on finding a way to alleviate food intolerance, which goes hand in hand with inflammation. During one of our phone chats, he told me that many people who came to see him about food intolerance also had issues with fertility. However, they didn't talk about it, because it's not what they went to see him for. He figured if he asked how many children they had, then it was like opening the floodgates to a dam. People were then more than happy to reveal their personal issues of why they didn't have children.

He would often hear how using ART methods not only broke the bank for couples but the emotional strain was devastating. The common story was IVF failed them, and they'd overextended themselves, used their entire savings or a big chunk of their superannuation trying to make it happen. It wasn't just over months, it was over years.

These kinds of responses led him to do more research into fertility. He found about 3 per cent of people who want to have children, can't have them due to food intolerance. He predicts by 2030 that this number will rise to about 50 per cent making it as he says, "the biggest health problem in the world and the biggest social problem, and economic problem."

While it takes sperm from a man and an egg from a woman to create a child, a lot of men refuse to consider they could be the problem; that they could be the cause of infertility.

As the professor shared with me, he said "there are two different species of human. One is called male and one is called female. The Australian male can't possibly have some imperfection like being unwell or not being fertile. I mean that is the ultimate insult."

Seedman was at least upfront with me about his infertility. It wasn't food intolerance related, though. His gun barrel had a blockage from birth. He was fortunate enough to already have twin teenage daughters through an ART procedure. Those tadpoles were torn from their cosy home in the epididymis, which is just above the testis. A small incision was made so a wad of sperm could be sucked out and used in IVF. To have more children would require more ART. More ART would require a sharp pointy thing attacking his crown jewels again. Of course, that was never, ever going to happen again.

To create a baby, not only does a woman have to be in her fertile window, healthy, stress-free and so on, but the sperm needs to be able to swim to the egg. With the natural response of the cervix being to fight off invaders, it can make for a frustrating mission. No matter how much you wish those little buggers would make it to that big, ripe and succulent egg, the vagina discharges the troops to slaughter these invaders.

Professor Hawkins told me that if a woman has food intolerance she has a very high concentration of immunoglobulin. Immunoglobulin binds to the sperm's membrane and really stops it progressing along into her ovaries. They become immobile and there is no way they can survive in a woman.

He spent a good chunk of his career honing natural formulations that are distributed not only around Australia but in a few locations around the world. For example, he found common plant foods, such as ginger and pineapple, were rich in unique natural enzymes making them ideal natural combatants in hostile environments.

Using his spice invader blend, the Professor has helped many women, who have attempted to become pregnant using failed ART. But like he told me, anyone who is going to conceive a child, no matter if they're fertile or not... needs a runway, a lead up. "Like a football player, you should train for at least three months before you run onto the field otherwise you get injured and that includes eating the correct food."

"All these people were not having success with IVF or any other means, so they had difficult situations where they had been written off. The most severe case of that was a lass who only had one ovary that was withered and had never ever produced a healthy egg." He told me she was around my age. She followed the professor's direction for the following months, and within the first month her "left ovary straightened up and produced a healthy egg for the first time in its life."

She then stayed on his program for another month and her other ovary produced a healthy egg. They then got her husband on the program as he was infertile, too. They had a healthy baby boy only twelve months later. "That child is now growing up a very healthy lad, and that came from a situation where the medical profession said the couple had no hope."

He says if you're at the stage where you just make a decision and want to immediately go for it, "go and get your body perfect for having that child. Don't sort of say, 'we're okay'."

The Professor spoke my language. I didn't really speak his with all the medical and scientific jargon, but I understood his message. His results spoke volumes. I got him. Along with his encouragement, I whisked half a teaspoon of his tuberous rhizome 'baby dust' formulation in a glass of water three times a day and sprinkled it, not so gingerly, over all my meals. This added another piece of armour in my path to pregnancy. I wanted strong eggs and a thriving picnic environment.

Looking for further reassurance that my own rogue plan was on track, I visited Joelene, a fertility naturopath. I met her at a spiritual expo and she instantly tapped into my vulnerability. She told me she worked from her home, so I made an appointment to meet with her the following week in the burbs. She worked towards the back of her house in a downstairs area. I walked through a side gate dodging all her drying laundry and entered through a back door. She was in the middle of housework but told me to take a seat as she needed to do a quick vacuum and then she'd be with me.

A few minutes later, she sat down at her desk, whisked her wiry grey hair back and pointed at a shelf displaying about a hundred different coloured bottles. She told me not to hesitate and choose four that immediately grabbed my attention. I picked out two similar bright pink ones with turquoise, then a sea blue one and finally a two-toned turquoise one then handed them to her. They seemed like potion bottles and I could only wonder what witchy spells she was going to brew up and sprinkle over me. If I was in luck, she would douse me in more baby dust.

I was told these were Aura Soma bottles and they would guide and support me towards well-being and self-awareness. It was of no surprise that she told me one bottle I had picked represented "the gift of being able to think 'outside of the box' and another reflected those who are seeking their true purpose."

This woman had no idea the extent of the wayward road I was travelling down. I certainly didn't know how to explain it to her. These bottles were totally in alignment with me. Oddly enough, they further assured me I was exactly where I was meant to be. I felt Joelene was another character along my yellow brick road who I was supposed to meet in my guerrilla pregnancy mission.

After my aura reading, she set me up in her backyard for a makeshift V-Steam. I can thank Gwyneth Patrow's outlandish Goop site for putting this treatment on my radar some years ago. Instead of catching up for a coffee or cocktail with my girlfriends, we would catch up for a little steam at a women's only bathhouse in Santa Monica. Quite a different set up to that of a suburban Brisbane backyard!

Joelene told me to strip off from the waist down, handed me a bunch of towels and directed me over to the holy chair in her backyard. When I say holy, I actually mean 'holey'. Her DIY open seated stool had just enough support for my legs and butt so my girly bits could hang loosely, uninterrupted over a mild steaming hot pot of herbal water. She plugged the slow cooker in, set it to a low heat with bunches of mugwort and rosemary slowly simmering below, and let me be.

I wrapped a towel around myself and wiggled out of my jeans, then tucked my tush through the hole. As I wrapped another towel around me to ensure no heat escaped, her landscaper moved from her front yard to the back. Here I was sitting half-naked over a steaming crock pot while it permeated the exterior of my vagina, as he hacked away at her Lilly Pilli hedge only metres from me. I shit you not.

I figured I've been in a few unusual positions of late, what was another?! I could not have made it up. For another thirty minutes he tended to the garden, and I tried relaxing as my vagina expanded and pulsated from the heat.

V-steams have a number of names. They're also known as yoni, bajos steams and chai-yoks. They're generally a very relaxing and nurturing steam. In my case, I'd say it wasn't so relaxing as much as it was quietly entertaining. I felt it was worth doing despite the unusual setup. The moist heat opens up the reproductive area bringing much-needed heat to the womb. The herbal water vapour carries the medicinal benefits of the plants, which gently increase blood flow to the uterus balancing hormone levels. I only hoped Mugwort was not infectious as I didn't feel it was conducive to my fertility mission. As two researchers out of New Zealand publicly declared on social media, "basically, it's sorcery for your vagina."

At 41 years-old, I was open to anything. Joelene wasn't quite yet done with me. Once my vagina 'Shallow Hal'd' on me, she got me on a massage table for a little uterus kneading to encourage more blood flow. Like I needed more blood flow down there, but I went with it. The massage is described as "deep pelvic organ visceral manipulative technique' and revitalises organs by bringing them to their natural and most optimal function.

For 20 minutes I laid back with a lavender pack over my eyes while her fist swirled, twirled and poked all my insides about. Finally four hours and a whole four hundred dollars later, I was released from the clutches of Joelene's magical ways to get on with my day. Once I got in my car I looked in the mirror. A puzzled expression looked back.

JUDGEMENT piped up, "Well that was a wee bit bizarre!" I slapped it down. "I'll have none of that. This is all part of my fertility force and I'm leading my charge. I'm open and available to whatever it takes—wizards, old aged but new age professors, white witches, aura spells and all!"

It was certainly a different approach to my weekly 5-minute chiro visits with the manipulation and adjustments, another tool I used to ensure my entire body, especially my pelvis, was correctly aligned so it was a clear runway for those swimmers to reach the egg.

As I drove home processing my woo-woo time with Joelene, I felt grateful to have found another person who also didn't buy into the medically infertile hogwash I had been told. Whatever she and the Professor handed out were the words I needed to hear. It was my candy and it gave me a high. They believed my body was very capable of holding a pregnancy and so did I. If women who are closer to their tombs can become mothers so late in the game, then surely my wholesome womb could, too.

I'd put myself under a microscope, but now it was time to throw the jiz shiz under it. I was dead set convinced that it was the sperm I had bought that had failed me. Not my eggs. Considering my "infertility issue" was purely based on my access to fresh sperm, of which I didn't have.

While sperm count is important, sperm motility is even more so. Before I proceeded with another IUI round or started IVF, I contacted my clinic to see if I could get a detailed overview of the sperm I had purchased. I wanted to know the breakdown of what I was being supplied with.

They refused to release this information to me, so I rang the cryobank that shipped it to them, but no one there was able to offer much information either. I called another cryobank who was able to help a little and conveniently sent me off to the WHO (World Health Organisation).

I found out that the samples I purchased had likely been spun before being frozen and shipped around the globe. That meant they had been spun twice before it was inserted into me. This didn't make a whole lot of sense to me as the prostaglandins had already been removed. I wondered if the second spin was to collect the sperm that couldn't be revived once they were thawed out?

Each vial I had purchased also only had a volume of half a mL with approximately 10 million sperm. While it only takes one super tadpole to crack open an egg, these figures were straight up awful. A typical healthy ejaculation should be between 2-5mLs and contain from 15 to 150 million sperm. That's a massive disparity which could potentially be the difference between having a baby and not having one.

It's information like this that would have swayed my decision on how I selected my anonymous donor. If I had known my chosen gentleman's sperm only just made it across WHO's baseline, I would certainly reconsider my donor selection. For me, I had presumed his low numbers and my old age weren't an optimal mix. Especially for an IUI procedure when you're paying the exact same dollar amount per vial; AND when each international semen vial costs over AU$1200 each.

I also found out that my twelve hundred bucks only reserved a vial; I didn't own the contents I'd paid for. At first, I thought perhaps it was because I couldn't own the container the contents came in, however, my research had me realise the donor has the right to withdraw consent at any given moment. They ultimately own the rights to their sperm. This is problematic if a woman purchases, I mean, reserves sperm vials, births a baby and then wants to use the remaining vials to try for a full biological sibling. It even means that any embryos created from the donor's sperm and a patient's eggs must be destroyed.

The jizzle shizzle gets worse. A recent study proves sperm counts aren't looking very promising in the western world. Very low parameters are considered 'normal' nowadays!

Volume > 1.5mL

Total Sperm > 39 million

Concentration Total ejac count > 15 million

Motility > 40%

Progressive Motility 32% (grade a+b)

Viable Sperm (Vitality) 58%

Morphology > 4%

These figures give a great indication of what you're working with, or perhaps not. And since conception for some can be a bit of a cat-and-mouse game in the known donor world, securing any sperm at all, can be in itself a feat.

In 2010, WHO changed the parameters measuring the health of men's sperm. Suddenly, some men were not considered as fertile as they once thought. Eleven years earlier in 1999, the minimum standard considered to be healthy sperm had to have a concentration of 20 million per mL with a 50 per cent motility, a 75 per cent vitality and 15 per cent morphology. That's quite a drop in numbers and very telling about the health of swimmers today. It's more like swimming downstream as opposed to up.

Australia imports their specimens from a few cryobanks and depending on what clinic you use will determine what bank they ship with. So, if you're using Monash and a friend is using Genea, chances are they will have different international donors as they will have imported from different cryobanks. Their paperwork, prices and processes can also vary.

When I was looking into using a clinic in Tasmania while I was there on business, they only had two viable donors, both of which were local Australians. They did not have access to international donors, and the wait on their two local donors had me placed at number thirteen in line.

## Mindset

If there is any kind of trauma, self-limiting beliefs, mental blocks or unstable memories, your path to having a baby can be affected as well. I believe that until I chose to put the final pin in my relationship with Ian, I was never truly open and ready to have a baby. I was still looking back, in fear of moving forward alone. It was keeping me in a flight holding pattern. I still had hope for some kind of reconciliation and I ultimately didn't want to move forward solo.

I was willing to settle for an unbalanced love-struggle relationship because I didn't want to get back out there in the big wide world to sell myself to secure another partner or let go of the fantasy life we were supposedly creating.

It was time to throw water on my inflamed thoughts. Turn down the volume on FEAR. Dislodge SHAME. Turn the page.

## Pregnancy Mantra

I can do this.
I'm a smart, resourceful woman.
I'm powerful, rational and responsible.
I have a body that was created to make and hold life.
I am deserving.
I'm worthy of a child or children choosing me.
My body wants this. I want this.

Chapter 12

# Gone Fishin'

*"The charm of fishing is that it is the pursuit of what is elusive
but attainable, a perpetual series of occasions for hope."*
*- John Buchan, politician*

## Seeking Assistance

"Single, 40-year-old,adrenal fatigued, career-focussed woman who missed the missed the 'memo for motherhood' seeks a strapping lad's fertile tadpoles.

Must be vertically and intellectually superior, sans chromosomal abnormalities, have abundant top-notch winning swimmers and be within close travelling-distance."

Feeling like I got my reproductive march-n-mojo on, I got the money back on my "reserved" donor vial for IVF and decided that going the (un) known donor route was a much better option for me. It felt right.

I knew this off the beaten track way outside of IVF existed, but I was hesitant to pursue it. It was the web's known donor or private donor option. It seemed to be the wild west of the donor world.

When I first landed on one of these sites at the beginning of my conception journey, I thought I had stumbled onto the fertility underbelly.

I was too fearful to take a really good peek around in case I found myself in some weird porn or body parts trafficking ring. But the idea did have some merit, so I filed it away and continued on my merry IVF and Tinder dating way.

Eighteen months on, and with both failed baby-making strategies behind me, the (un)known/private donor alternative surfaced again. I was still very curious about this route but was hesitant about its safety and the more intricate and complex ramifications that came with it. I nabbed it out of my brains storage compartment and decided to break it open, take the plunge and see if it really was really feasible.

I mean, honestly, could it really be that shady? After all, lesbians have been using these kinds of means for decades. JUDGEMENT along with DOUBT was hovering, though. I could feel them intensely, but I managed to squish them back into their little box and continued with my online exploration.

It took just a few taps on my keyboard for my monitor to display dozens of men from all over the world happily offering their free baby batter to wannabe mamas. I realised they weren't all the whack jobs and freaks that I had presumed they would be, i.e. the types of people I prefer to avoid. Many were men that I'd chat to if I were in a bar, sit next to in a movie theatre or fill an empty seat beside them on a train. They were everyday men of all different shapes, colours and sizes. I realised they were just like us everyday women who were desperately seeking semen.

Having marinated over this back alley channel for so long, and now having broken away the negative thoughts I had towards this avenue, pushing JUDGEMENT out of the way, the idea of heading in this direction didn't seem so aberrant now.

In fact, using semen from someone that required no relationship labour and wouldn't financially break me was gaining more green lights than reds...more ticks than crosses. Rather than studying pages of a donor's profile, that may or may not be true, and scrutinising thumbnail photos that only pixelated when zoomed in, I could actually check this human out myself, have a real-time conversation and even get current medical records. This all made insanely good sense. Hallelujah, I could skip all the dating 'let's get to know each other' chit-chat and long-term relationship rollercoaster bullshit and just discuss the ins and outs of making a baby pronto.

Armed with a referral to a radiologist for both a HSG and a HyCoSy, up-to-date STI and AMH tests, a backup prescription for Clomid if needed, two different OPK's, following the Ovia app, an AI kit, communications journal, monitoring cervical fluid, tracking days, taking my vitamins, having consulted with various natural therapists and fulfilling my counselling obligation, I felt I was now ready to stop surfing for swimmers and take a deep dive in.

I had done my homework and as far as I believed, I really had thrown the net out far and wide. I had scrolled through different donor websites, donor sperm FB Groups, donor FB pages, read news articles and blogs on a donor registry. I looked at the viability of shipping semen, using international donors, and looked at what other clinics were offering so I could get a really good lay of the land. Now with a great understanding of this wayward landscape, I was truly ready to reel in a free-roaming sword fish.

I signed up on a paid known donor site and set up another account with a free one. Along with a recent legitimate photo, I threw this plea wide out into the sea:

"I'm a 5'6 tall, single, 41 yo and my background is in TV producing. I'm also currently setting up an online business to build passive income and support a flexible lifestyle.

I see myself as a "global citizen" having just returned to Queensland after ten years of living in the US. I'm a bit of an earth warrior and don't always comply with the norm. I've travelled the planet with entrepreneurs learning and seeing how we can be better and do more. And this is a lifestyle I will continue with especially as I have global friends who I call family.

It wasn't my plan to be single but my three-year relationship crumbled and I was left at 40 not holding the baby (so to speak). We tried so hard to make it work but we just weren't on the same page. So we let each other go and rather than be a victim I've decided to search out other ways to be a parent.

I also don't believe it's fair to go out in the world pressing my agenda while I try to meet the love of my life. It's too much pressure and would have me end up in something with someone for the wrong reason. So I've had to accept that I now have to find another path first to travel down then be open for that love to come.

Unfortunately, stats more than show not all relationships are everlasting. Therefore I would rather meet someone while I'm living true to me, fulfilled and happy. It changes the energy of that union and I want to be with someone who can function 'intradependently' with me.

I'm a strong woman having left home at 17 and leaving Perth for Sydney at 21. I moved to the US when I was 30. I put my career first and dated lots of wrong or wrong time guys....perhaps I was never ready until now? Being back in Oz is very grounding and I have so much support here. A clinic declared me socially infertile and after three IUI attempts, I am now deemed medically infertile.

The only path they suggest for me is IVF with drugs which just doesn't resonate with me. I've been liaising with a medical professor and I'm 100 per cent in good health. Sure my age doesn't help, but as I can't get any real info on the semen I purchase through IVF I can't help but think their system is flawed. It's not a way that energetically fits with me....so here I am!!

Ideally, I am looking for the generosity of one super kind man to assist me in my motherhood quest. Physically tall, fit, healthy, local to SE Qld although I am willing to travel, intelligent and willing to share recent medical records with me, or will work with me on getting those done.

Most of all I would like someone who is on the same page about bringing a soul into this world. We can figure that out once we connect. Thanks in advance for reading my profile, I look forward to chatting with you, and thanks so much for offering to assist women who too need you!"

I had no time to waste and figured if I wrote a message that was true for me then I'd have a greater chance of clinching a solid candidate or two. I then started perusing through donor profiles to see if any words or pictures struck a chord with me. Many were vague, photoless or geographically challenging, but there were a few that gave me hope. I wasn't sure if this really was the way forward but figured it was worth the hundred bucks to find out.

By the next day, I had received some bites but none that deeply resonated with me. I was so grateful that there were potential baby daddy's out there, though, and that they were now just a yay or nay away.

One gentleman by the name of Lucas wrote to me. He only shared one photo, which was of him facing away from the camera holding hands with his two children. He was keen for me to email him outside the platform which I swiftly questioned. My response requested that he divulge a bunch of medical details along with his intentions first. He responded straight back with answers and his mobile number inviting me to give him a call. This all became very real and I was a step closer to perhaps having the chance to be a mum. I freaked out and promptly got off the site.

As my eyes locked onto a spot through the window opposite me, my inner dialogue was going head to head as I tried to make sense of what I was doing. My brain literally burst open with all the shady 'what ifs'.

What if he just wants sex? What if he has diseases? What if he's a weirdo? What if he's the guy that has long unwashed head and body hair, no teeth and is a hunchback that goes to the local derelict bar every day and sinks his entire pension check into the pokies?

My apprehension fuelled an all-out clash of my emotions. JUDGEMENT and SHAME didn't hold back spitting up one of Ian's slap downs that he threw at me in one of our many previous heated conversations, "If you randomly fuck some guy in a bar to make a baby we'll never be together." Ian was adamant he wasn't interested in bringing up or having relations with a bastard child.

HOPE was fading fast. She cried out, "Sure this path can perhaps be seedy but you're searching for seeds! Seeds bear fruit so they can be fruitful too...you don't throw out the whole apple cart because one piece of fruit is bad. And you don't even know if they're rotten, you're letting them psych you out."

JUDGEMENT threw back, "What kind of man goes on a website offering free sperm? A freak, that's who!"

SHAME chimed in, "This is idiotic. You're a loser that you can't get a man and you have to resort to this. How embarrassing! What happened to you? You were someone who could have had it all! Imagine what all your friends think of you!"

I felt like I had just landed back at square one. Not only did I have my own fears, concerns and shame to contend with, but I was also carrying the load of others too. And I would learn about more a little further down the track.

I realised pretty quickly that donor profiles were easy to categorise and through my observations I was able to compile a character profile list:

## Private Donor Types:

- Wolf - Preys on vulnerable women desperate to have a child just to have sex. These are the creeps! He is likely to be married and uses donoring as an excuse to get sex or refuse to pay for it so use this avenue. It's highly likely he has multiple accounts and profiles. Stay aware!

- One Time Wonder - Similar to wolves in that he just wants to have sex with as many people as possible. He will have NI with a recipient once and never come back to help again despite sex being available next month.

- Fraudster Flake - Inconsistent, only responds randomly, carrot danglers, disinterested and wastes time and energy. Run!

- The Progenitor - Uses a fake name and profile as they're unsure

- or distrusting of the legal system. Don't want to create a public spectacle, communicates privately. His behaviour can come across as suspicious even if he is not.

- Pronor - Professional Donor. Easy, efficient, knowledgeable, and will work with you to help you conceive wherever you are in the world if you pick up the bill. May have assisted in the conception of a few children or hundreds.

- Non-Discriminatory Pleaser - He is open and readily available. Will hand over his seeds to anyone. He believes he is serving a higher purpose but is mostly doing it to satisfy his ego. Or God.

- Testy's - Not using his "testes" but testing the waters. He sits on sites for months or years indecisive or inactive. He really isn't sure about donating.

- Green Donors - New to the site, unprepared, not tested. Can take months to get them donor ready which can be incredibly frustrating.

- The "Uncle" - Hasn't had kids and would love to participate in co-parenting or at the very least share his seed.

- The Private Benefactor - Family man, single or married and active in wanting to help the right person or couple because he can. Likely to only donate to ten women or less.

- Diversity Donor - Likes to assist all nationalities.

- Infertile/Sterile Donor - A serial donor who is delusional. Believes he can assist even though the lack of results proves otherwise. Can prey on the vulnerable and desperate but truly believes he can help.

- Mr Selective - Will only donate to a specific type of recipient. Has a very high standard and only a lucky few fit his donation criteria - financial, physical attributes, health, lifestyle values, marital status or gender persuasion.

- Eugenics Donator - Believes his seed will improve the human race.

- Addict - Sets out as a regular donor then fast becomes a pronor/serial donor. He is obsessed and addicted to the rush of his successes, the thrill of helping people and being forever applauded by recipients for his good will. Likely to help hundreds of women.

- Voyeur - Uses a fake profile as camouflage so he (or she) can just snoop about. Could be a donor with multiple aliases, a spy such as a suss donor wife or an ex-partner stalking people.

*Green and Testy donors (are also progenitors) can be family men married or not, or young singles, who just want to assist one family or single woman.

That's when I joined the Sperm Donation Australia FB group. Thankfully Adam Hooper, (SDA Adam) the admin of the group, was able to bridge the gap and guide me into the "dark" side with ease. Surprisingly, the dark side was a whole lot brighter than I could have imagined. Seedier too—in a favourable way!

Before allowing me into the group, Adam sniffed me out a little. He asked me who I was and why I was trying to join his group. While I was responding, he researched me wondering if I was a journo just snooping around. I assured him I wasn't and I was desperately in need of seed.

Our online chat lasted an hour. It then continued into the following few days. He answered all my questions and assured me that all my hesitations and thoughts were just like every other woman's searching for sperm. I was so relieved! I also felt like I had landed upon a community of like-minded folk. It felt safer than the other sites I was on.

Adam gets that feedback all the time. It's probably because he manages the group responsibly. Upon requesting access, pending members receive a comprehensive message introducing himself and outlining the rules he's established for the group.

He lets people know that he doesn't accept just anybody. They must be able to answer his list of questions about giving or receiving donations among other qualifying questions. He attempts to weed out, well, the weeds. He tries to ensure ALL new members are aware of the criminal ramifications associated with knowingly passing on STIs and accepting payment for giving/receiving human fluids. Knowing all too well that people have different parenting views, he requests all to refrain from vilifying anyone publicly.

I hadn't seen such a thorough donor profile until I saw Matt C's posted on the group's newsfeed. I liked that he'd made so much effort, answering so many questions upfront.

Later, when I spoke to him for information for this book, I asked why he wrote such a lengthy piece. He told me he created a comprehensive post "as a way of not wasting each other's time trying to dig around to get that information." That's right, this ain't dating baby!

His post also works as a filtering tool to eliminate people who don't respond to the way he thinks such a post deserves. "I put so much in there that if I get a message from someone in there that goes, "I want a donor will you help me?" Then it kind of goes like, "Well, why would I go to all this effort, and continue to, if someone isn't going to respect that and put in some effort."

## This was his original posting:

*"I'm a 30 yo donor from Brisbane. I've been lucky enough to help 2 women become pregnant so far from AI donations (1 is having a boy, the other doesn't know yet) and I'm looking to continue that.*

*I decided to become a donor because of the immense, positive impact it can have on someone's life, because it requires relatively little from me for the impact that it makes, and because there seems to be a big demand for donors at the moment. I'm just trying to do something good for someone else in the hope that they pay it forward and help someone else one day when they can.*

*A little about me:*

*My father is from Denmark and my mother's family is Australian for a few generations, but can be traced back to Scottish & German*

*At 188 cm tall, I am the tallest person in my extended family (though my older brother and some of my cousins come close). My mum is a shorty though, only pushing about 155cm :P*

*I recently finished a BSc and a Project Management certification and am looking to start an MBA in the new year. I am also qualified to teach people how to fly planes.*

*I played the piano as a child (and am looking to take it back up again) and used to write/produce a little trance music a while back. I got a few dj gigs around the country, but mostly in Perth where I grew up.*

*I have been an avid bodybuilder for the past 7 years and have taken up AFL this year for the first time since I was 13. I lead a generally healthy lifestyle, but do enjoy a few drinks socially.*

*I have 1 older and 1 younger brother, no nephews or nieces, and a fairly even distribution of males & females amongst my cousins.*

*I have no family history of illnesses (though I do have rather flat feet and did have braces as a child, so did my mum).*

*Both of my parents are still alive. My mum is 58 and my dad is 65. I only have 1 grandmother left and no grandfathers.*

*If there is anything else you would like to know, please feel free to ask.*

*I am currently focusing on AI (specimen cup & syringe method), but will consider NI or clinic based on circumstances. I have a contract in place that I have been using with all recipients so far that basically says that 100% of parental rights and responsibilities belong to the recipients and their family, and that I have none. I am happy for the child to know who I am and meet me (either as a child or once they turn 18), but it may only be done by prior arrangement with the recipient and myself. I do request that I at least have a photo and some basic info from the birth, and would like to be sent updates occasionally (birthdays or special occasions/achievements/etc).*

*I usually come to the recipient, either to their home or to a hotel room they have booked, for the donation, and I am happy to discuss travel outside of Brisbane, as long as I am not out of pocket at all. My last STD check was in mid April and it came back all clear (which I can provide you copies of). I am happy to get another one in the near future as required and will be getting checked every 6 months at a minimum. I am also looking at getting a fertility test done for sperm count and motility, but no solid dates are booked in as yet. I am happy to make multiple donations per cycle and donate for multiple cycles. I am also happy to donate for multiple children to a single family so that they are all genetically related, if you wish.*

*Thanks for taking the time to read my post—I know it's a bit of an essay. I just prefer to cover as much info up front as possible. As such, I would request that you do the same if you pm me.*

*My main concern is that the child grows up in a healthy and safe environment, where all their needs are provided for. Any information you can provide about yourself and your partner to support this would be greatly appreciated and makes the whole process much easier for all parties involved. I also strongly prefer that everyone meets face-to-face before starting donations, just to ensure that everyone is as comfortable as possible with each other before we begin.*

*Thanks again, and I look forward to chatting with some of you soon."*

I think it's fair to assume that if Matt C ain't getting the same love back with a worthy and eloquent response to match that, then there's not much chance of getting any fresh taddies (tadpoles) from Matty.

There are some known donors who don't want to get bogged down in the personal story of recipients; they want it to be transactional. Short and sweet. A less-is-more kind of deal. I was bringing a child into the world so for me, the man I created that child with, needed to be able to offer more than a few words.

Feeling somewhat in better company and more comfortable with progressing forward, I felt confident in making some moves. Since this was my mission, I didn't just put out a plea and think it was enough to secure a donor. To get the outcome I so desired I had to work for it. And so I did.

Surprisingly, they were quite a decent bunch of blokes who also came with good testimonials from Adam. I made a list of my top ten donors and then wrote to the first five through the FB group while simultaneously chatting to a few potential donors on the paid and unpaid sites.

Ding dong! Four potential donor-daddies-to-be responded to my message. One was in Ireland, one fought fires in South Australia, another was a married man in Canberra and another was a 22-year-old party kid in Perth who was just dipping his big toe in.

I hit up the number one guy on my list first who was a spunky firefighter in South Australia. We dialogued a bit, but it was immediately obvious he wasn't in it for the right reasons. He only wanted to discuss sexual escapades and was aloof when it came to nailing him down for honest responses. I put that fire out about thirty minutes after we engaged and smudged my room with a big chunk of sage. I scratched hunky number two off the list, too, due to his geographical location.

There was no way I was flying to Ireland on a hope and a prayer. Besides, there was plenty of fish to catch closer to home. Perth party boy seemed ideal, however, as I found out a 'play hard' partier. He was a green donor, had not completed any medical tests, needed to get off the Gunga and cigarettes and minimise his social drinking. Fair to say, he was going to be some work. Work translated into time. Time I couldn't hold out for. And I really didn't want to mother my donor...just his offspring.

The Canberran was number five on my list, but after our Facetime chat, he climbed the ladder to take out the number one spot. He and his feminist wife decided they wanted to help out a family or two. Both were smart, well-travelled and had the same values about parenting as I did. They were the type of people I could see myself moving forward with and stay connected to post-conception. The perfect benefactor!

Unfortunately, due to an unexpected personal situation, they had to delay donating for a few months. It was a big blow for me too, but I didn't let it stop me remaining open and continuing with my search. This known donor pool was filled with options, and I was confident it wouldn't be long for another good catch to come along.

I felt much more assertive and comfortable in this arena now. I even had the courage to write back to Lucas from the paid donor site. He hadn't been online in a while, but I hoped he'd receive a message notification. While I waited for him to get back to me, a donor from the FB group contacted me.

Now that I had found my stride, I immediately asked if he was willing to take our chat to second base. He fast became my Interstate Man Of Mystery with the killer radio voice. An FB pronor with a few successful inseminations, including two recent births, under his belt. He had my attention and was now my number one pick.

IMOM (Interstate Man of Mystery) and I stayed in touch through one ovulation cycle. The next was not long on the horizon. I needed to make a decision. Wait for Lucas to respond, keep talking to other potential donors or seize the moment?

My inner critics raised their voices again.

FEAR and DOUBT: He could be a freak!

BIO CLOCK: Tick, tock, tick, tock.....

ASPIRATIONS, HOPE, LOVE: This is the window—the one you climb through not jam shut!

I kicked FEAR and DOUBT to the curb. I seized the moment.

*Chapter 13*

# Mr. Stork

*"All in all, after just a couple of months and a few discarded swimmers due to not meeting the legal requirements, I got an agile one on the hook that fit my criteria."*
*- Hayley Hendrix, HuffPost Blog, November 2017*

*"All human beings have three lives: public, private, and secret."*
*- Gabriel García Márquez, novelist*

I WASN'T LOOKING FOR A life partner; I was looking for a donor. For me, they were two very different people. After 25 years of dating and seemingly not being able to get it right, I decided to focus on the attributes I wanted for a child not what I wanted for me.

IMOM broke down my own uneducated thoughts I had towards donors and the JUDGEMENT others had poisoned me with. While I didn't know his name, how he moved, what he wore or what he smelled like, we talked so much that I felt as though I knew him. Like my other senses led the way because my eyes were less involved in the investigation process.

Yes, we swapped photographs, but learning about one another primarily through auditory means, allowed me to make a decision based on other important factors.

What was uncomfortable dinner conversation with Seedman, came with ease with IMOM. We had connected with one intention in mind and that was to make a baby. There was no dancing around the topic.

Once we made that pact, I aptly renamed IMOM, Mr Stork; and our donor romance officially began. This 'domance' was the phase where we engaged in all the nitty gritty conversation before committing to a full-blown donorship (donor relationship) which would include the insem and beyond.

This was how it played out online:

*FB Group: You accepted Mr Stork's request*

*Mr Stork: Hi Hayley welcome to the Sperm Donors:) Group. Are you looking for a donor or just having a look at how it all works?*

*Hayley: Seeking a donor via AI.*

*Mr Stork: Yeah no worries. Do you have a co parent profile at all too?*

*Hayley: Where are you located and how are you looking at donating?*

*Mr Stork: I am taking you are strictly looking for AI. AI is fine. I have done it in the past. I have had 3 successes now.*

*Hayley: Congratulations on your successes!*

*Hayley: Yup. I want clear boundaries.*

*Hayley: So I'm interested, why are you a donor?*

*Mr Stork: I was at university at 19 and was asked by Monash IVF to be a donor.....they had a stall at the UNI......and I thought I was way too young to decide.....fast forward to 4 years ago.....I found out I have a extreme sperm count......and good genes.......then my partner and I broke up so I thought why not help others.......so it's been a long journey to get to this point.*

*I don't put pictures on my profile as I have my own child to a former relationship.....and I don't want my own child to see I am a donor on the internet.*

*Hayley: Are you straight? Het/gay/bi?*

*Mr Stork: Yes very boringly heterosexual*

*Mr Stork: so question for you why are you a recipient??*

*Hayley: Well it wasn't my plan to be single but my three year on/off relationship crumbled and I was left nearing 40 not holding the baby (so to speak). I don't believe it's fair to go out in the world pressing my agenda only to end up a couple of years later in a custody battle over a child I so desperately wanted. I'd rather meet that special someone as a package deal—while I'm living true to me, fulfilled and happy as a mother operating on my own terms.*

*Mr Stork: Spot on.*

*Hayley: So while that relationship works its way into my world, I'm continuing on my path without forcing someone onto mine.*

*Mr Stork: Good call......*

*Hayley: Unfort time is against me. So I've had to make some decisions I wouldn't ordinarily make. I must see recent STI test and semen analysis before progressing. Ideally progressive motility is of utmost importance!*

*Mr Stork: Hmm I agree*

*Hayley: So you're tall. Slim. Strong features. Smart. Kind? A person I don't mind connecting with in the future. AI only. All the bits in the right places? You seem ideal!*

*Mr Stork: right........real donors will have semen testing done......and have good knowledge about the whole reproductivity of women and men. I can send you a picture but is just for OK? If I am too Italian looking I will understand.*

*I am a donor not a man looking for sex ......I am not an ugly man........ having said that I would not do heaps of AI at your age......either switch to sex or fresh IUI if you can find a clinic to do it...for me its get the pregnancy happening...I take supplements to help the count...I am treating it in a professional manner. So far 2 first goes have gotten pregnancy with AI...and one took four goes AI...so its working. By the way not bragging just being up front. I have had the genetic screen done the clinics do. cystic fibrosis, karyotype, Fragile X syndrome (FXS) don't carry them.*

*Hayley: Thank you for being honest.*

*Mr Stork: 9-11 mL per ejac..it's huge. Most is 2.5-5*

*Hayley: My iuis were 0.5mLs. I have been very frustrated.*

*Mr Stork: and half of that was sperm cryoprotectant*

*Hayley: That's why I decided to search out a "fresh" new option.*

*Mr Stork: I like the way you are rolling about all this..........and your knowledge of male fertility is a massive tick.......and I would love to help you beat the clock.*

Certainly not Tinder or first date chat! For me, it was so refreshing to be able to engage in such banter from the get-go. I felt like the dance was over, and I could just book in a date to try for a baby opposed to a date for a dinner to dance around the conversation.

The photos he shared early on with me were, to be honest, not exceptional marketing materials. One was an old black and white pic from when he was in his twenties and another had his gigantic green eyes concealed under sunglasses. There were no smiles either, which was disappointing to not be able to peruse. My instant thought was he had either banged up teeth or was missing a few which would be a total turn off for me. There's nothing quite like a sparkle in someone's eyes and wide smile to draw you in. So ladies, ensure you get images of those pearly whites and eyes!

In any case, he too had me hooked. Our text chat elevated to an old-fashioned voice one, where we continued to dig down and ask those 'what would normally take months to ask' type awkward q's and eyeball his test results.

Turned out, Mr Stork was actually a fellow middle-aged but unbelievably rich man. He was a flippin' billionaire! I was beside myself with excitement that I'd snagged him. Finding this information out merely in minutes sent me into a tailspin.

If any there was a time I was proud to be referred to as a gold digger then this would be it! These types of women were prolific in Hollywood and watching them burn my male friends in bars was a fun but cruel weekend past time.

For instance, my friend Glenn on one occasion gave out a flirty "g'day" to a woman waiting in line next to him at a busy bar on Sunset Blvd. She responded by asking how much money he earned.

Of course his knee jerk response was to tell her to "fuck off" which basically just reaffirmed him that all LA (hot) women were shallow money grabbing bitches. Ian also had a stack of stories about actresses he dated before meeting me. One girl shamelessly asked if he would grab groceries on his way over to take her out and another if he could pick up her rent that month. Both were first (and last) dates! I couldn't ever imagine being as brazen as those women. Until now! I was thrilled to find out Mr Stork's trouser pockets were loaded.

While his net worth probably wouldn't have impressed any of those young women, I knew the value of his stocks. His uberous sperm could impregnate a nation. The best thing of all is that his account was always topped up. Kind of like a money tree that always grew cash.

His testis kept filling the silos with more seeds. This was a 'jackpot' like no other and he truly was a 'seedman'.

This, along with his pro-approach swayed the vote for me. He knew loads about women's fertility and reproduction, which oddly impressed me. I didn't think a man just on the prowl for sex would engage in that type of conversation. The dialogue I'd had with the hunky South Australian firefighter proved that. They were two very different interactions even though they were using the same platform. Having said that, what's wrong with a guy offering to assist in child-making enjoying himself? If you feel the same way, what's the problem with that? I was driven by the outcome so was wanting someone up to speed and well versed so he could join me where I already was on this path and then travel at my pace.

Just as STI testing is mandatory through IVF clinics, I also had Mr Stork provide me with these test results. He showed me blood tests that included full blood count, blood group, HIV 1 and 2, Hepatitis B, Hepatitis C, Syphilis, Human T-lymphotropic virus, type I and II and Cytomegalovirus. Urine tests for Gonorrhoea, Chlamydia as well as a full semen analysis.

I also didn't want to waste time with a sterile man. And believe me, there are a few of them who may actually be in it for the right reasons but can't produce children no matter how convinced they think they can. I cover this further in the CONtroversy chapter.

I was acutely aware of this issue as I manoeuvred my way along my merry semen path. However, there's no way I'd consider using a donor without ensuring his semen was in tip-top shape before even embarking on a domance.

During our conversations, it was very clear Mr Stork was a donor combo. He had Pronor and Progenitor ways with a little Mr Selective thrown in. Combined, they were both a positive and a negative. Positive in that his sperm actually worked, but a little concerning as I personally find it hard to grock the idea that a man would possibly want to sow his seed across a village. He assured me that was not his intention and he certainly wasn't competing for the title of Super(se)man, but I only had his word to go by. I knew I couldn't even get this reassurance using sperm in a clinic. So, if I wanted to do this, then I'd have to accept that I have no control over someone else's decisions. I had already resigned myself that my child would be genetically linked with others during my clinic counselling.

It came with this pathway. A handful of half-siblings I could get my head around. Thirty, fifty, one hundred, just seemed too big. Too much. Well, at this early stage of my known donor journey anyway. Mr Stork had not only offered to assist me, but he could also offer me more than sixty times the baseline sperm count quantity that WHO recommends. His numbers were beyond impressive and they totally assured me—he was Mr Right, right now.

Mr Stork provided me with his recent semen analysis that consisted of:

- Total Progressive Motility
- Morphology percentage
- Total Sperm Count
- Semen Volume

I reflected back on what the professor told me about how Australian men refuse to consider they might have a real illness, or be infertile, as it's seen as emasculating to them. He also told me women were used to being checked out as they were more likely to have lumps and bumps with issues, so it's only been fairly recent that men have opened themselves up for testing, which is why we now know that around 40 per cent of infertility can be traced to the blokes. That's almost half, which demonstrates the important role healthy sperm plays.

I was thrilled that my donor was abreast of this. He took his health seriously, took a daily vitamin, ate a healthy diet (according to him), didn't smoke or drink alcohol and played a weekly team sport. Research shows that poor eating habits and regular consumption of alcohol, for instance, can lower the quality and quantity of sperm, making conception more difficult. Eating healthily not only boosts sperm quality and quantity, it assists in increasing the chances of conceiving a healthy child.

His sperm numbers combined with his physical attributes, availability, location, clean medical records, humour, compassion along with the added bonus of connecting with one another at the perfect time and his providing the mentoring I needed to forget the pain of the past and focus on the now, had me grade him an A.

This was different to my friend Carmen, who found making that final decision on who that donor would be quite emotional. She called her best friend and had a long conversation about her selection process. "We talked long and hard about the impacts of nature versus nurture and how that influences a child's life and future." For her, deciding on what donor semen she was going to use was, "more emotional than going through each unsuccessful cycle of IVF. Choosing a donor meant making THE decision on WHO my future child was going to be."

Since Mr Stork had the same objective in mind, it eliminated so many pain points for me. He cared about who the mother of this child would be and how that would influence the way the child would be brought up, and therefore, who they could become. I felt as though I had someone who really got me and my circumstance and was willing to work not just for me, but alongside me. He knew there was little space for error and what the high price of missing a cycle really was. With potentially only twelve chances a year and egg quality probably declining each month, it was imperative I wasn't being fucked around.

This is where it gets tricky with donors. It's illegal in most places around the globe to pay for sperm so they're working for YOU for FREE to assist YOU so YOU can achieve YOUR goal. Not necessarily theirs.

Maybe theirs is to sire a city, but more than likely it's not. You'll know it if they are! Expecting them to be available to assist you throughout your ovulation cycle is a big ask especially when they could be potentially needed to assist you for months, even a year (or more), and possibly for multiple pregnancies. The right donor understands this and will be flexible to meet your needs over these days.

Mr Stork had already donated to a couple of women and had his own criteria for who he would assist, which was, obviously, someone who was really wanting a child and had a legitimate story. I guess I must have passed through that hoop. He said he really liked "helping older women who are trying to beat that clock." Thank goodness for that! Tick. He also prefers women who "have done their homework and he doesn't have to teach them about their ovulation cycles." I certainly did that!

He said that he found it frustrating how many women he spoke with who didn't have basic reproduction education. During one of our earlier conversations he told me, "A lot of women don't have this knowledge...so opposed to chatting about the donor stuff and their situation, I have to go explain all the basic stuff, like how a cycle works."

He also found this kind of basic banter dispiriting. Like these women weren't really making an effort or hadn't fully comprehended the enormity and complexity of it all. "I want clear indication of what they want. I don't do wavering. If there's some wavering, I won't move forward with them." This sentiment also goes both ways!

Despite primarily being driven by sheer desperation, Mr Stork didn't shy away from the task at hand. He remained calm and committed to the mission. I was overcome with a wide range of emotions because at the end of the day this was a very out of the box thing for me to do. It could even be considered to be an explicit jiz jaunt. So while I was hell bent on fossicking for my piece of gold, we wanted to keep it as a fun, light hearted and exciting experience.

Our domance was swiftly solidified and before I knew it, my ovulation cycle one was upon us. I felt we were ready to take the plunge. I'd been monitoring an ovulation cycle app on my phone as well as counting my days. I pulled out the OPK's (ovulation predictor kits) that I had stored and pooled all the info together to see how I was travelling in this window. I was pretty sure it was day fourteen, which meant that my egg was almost ready to be released or perhaps it already had.

I contacted Mr Stork to find out what his plans were that night and over the next couple of days. He said he would be around and available should I choose to move forward this cycle. As I had endured a two- month cooling off period after my failed IUIs, I was eager to get going. I felt this route was right for me. I was more than ready, just shy of being overly cooked, to get a bun in my oven.

As the hours rolled by, the two OPK's gave me different results. One app showed I was in prime time for fertile slime insemination and my day count seemed accurate, the other had me doubting my target time, but I was sure my count was right. I called Mr Stork to ask for his advice on whether or not I should chance a plane ride down to semen, I mean, see him. He said he would be wherever I needed him to be.

I was at Kim's house bringing her up to speed and she assured me my math was accurate. That the pee on stick OPK was AOK and my ovu app was AG (all good). I made the decision that if I could get on a flight in the next two hours then it was a G.O. Chez got me on a flight, Kim shoved me in her car and drove me to the airport and the next thing I knew…

Here I am on a plane heading south to meet Mr Stork in the flesh to create a baby. So, who is my Mr Stork? While I know him, I don't know him.

*Chapter 14*

# Y?

WHY DO GUYS DONATE? *I* mean, what's in it for them? I asked a few what their intentions were, so I could gain some deeper insight. Turns out there really are some good guys out there. Yup, I said it again. Until recently, JLM ran the Sperm Donor FB Group with Adam. His reasons for donating came about from an experience he had in his childhood. "When I was eleven-years-old I had ruptured appendix and peritonitis and someone saved my life with blood donation and so I was paying it back."

Having had a couple of successes having children of his own as well as a couple of losses, he felt he could empathise with people who endure infertility. "That desperate need for children and that loss of not having them...being empathetic and being a Christian and knowing I should contribute to my fellow man, so I did."

When Christian and Juan, a gorgeous gay couple living in Sydney became parents with the assistance of an egg donor and surrogate, they felt they wanted to give back. So they joined the FB donor group to help out a select handful of women. "We felt in debt with karma. We were so grateful and thankful for the gift that they had given us that we thought we had to give back something to the world and humanity."

Similarly to JLM, Chris, who is a lawyer, chose to be a private donor. I mean he's been a long time blood and registered organ donor, so why not? He had been donating to a clinic but felt he could help more people outside of one as the law has restrictions in place for AI. He sees this as a chance to help couples who desperately want to have children, but who can't for medical reasons. "I saw a one page advertisement pinned to a notice board at university when I left school, and it stayed in my mind for years afterwards because my family has a long history of living to a very old age, and we are a family without any serious medical problems and that is the gift that I felt that I should be giving, and wanted to give, to couples who can't have children on their own."

For Adam, it was his wife that put donoring on his radar. She was working with someone who was looking for a donor, which put the idea into his head. He looked at his two children, and he "saw how cool they were for me and thought how cool it would be for me to help other people."

Of the many things that irk Adam about clinics, its how they mislead people. They can't guarantee the capped number of offspring produced per donor even though this is what they tell women. That same sperm sold in clinics still gets sold overseas by clinics which has their own family quotas. Cryobanks even ship the same sperm specimens direct to customers for home inseminations. The result—hundreds of kids born out of the same DNA. It's not foolproof and not even uncommon for women who use donor sperm to fall pregnant and not inform the doctors of their pregnancies. Their system too is wholly based on trust and this is just one of many gaping holes in the fertility industry system. It's frightening knowing that a handful of fertility doctors have switched out donor's semen for their own and have gotten away with it for decades.

There are some men out there who are out to plant their seed as far and wide as can be. I guess it gives them some kind of celebrity and they feel as though they truly are doing good in the world. While it's easy to criticise them, there's also the flip side—they're actually helping people who really want a baby.

Men such as Simon Watson and Mitch Kennedy in the UK, Joe Donor and Matt Stone in the US and Ed Houben who's hailed as 'Europe's most virile man' have assisted many women with babies.

Between them, they have created hundreds of humans and these guys all pretty well known in donorland. They can all be easily searched and found online along with other well-known donors. Ed, who apparently has over 100 donor children, began donating to a clinic in 2002 but now donates the 'natural' way God intended, according to an article in the Daily Mail. For US$180 you can receive sperm specimens within the USA via the post with Joe who has, along with Matt (just recently retired) fathered 250 kiddies between them.

Simon also donates via the post charging a hundred quid for his pot of potential joys or as it states on his website, you can meet him in "a public place like a supermarket car park or petrol station.....you name it. Including your own premises." Mitch has helped the least families out of these donors to date, and only hands over his jiz in a bottle to selected women who are mostly lesbians.

Perhaps they have the Eugenic syndrome? It's the decision of a woman if she chooses to use a man's sperm that's been used to create an extraordinarily large progeny. Clinics can't really even monitor this either (unless it's publicised) as some men donate to them and to women at their own free will. Personally, I just think of the kiddies and how that impacts them.

Jim Smith thought all women looking to have a baby would be really nice and wonderful and it would be a warm experience for all. He was taken aback when this wasn't the case. I guess the types of people donors engage with depends on where they advertise their 'altruistic' services. There are a few dodgy donor sites out there, just as there are dating ones that attract a low-end mentality.

Unlike Simon Watson who is happy to assist women in public places, Jim is not. He found himself at the receiving end of a few requests that were plain gross. "Can I meet you in a carpark? Can I jack off in a toilet at a petrol station? Can you help me have a baby for Centrelink (Government payments)? And I had two lesbians tell me that no man can masturbate in their house so I'd have to masturbate elsewhere, put it in the cup and bring it in."

He used to publicly display a profile with a few photos, including some from his childhood, on a paid donor site. Once he received these types of hideous requests, he removed his honest and transparent profile pictures and created an alias. He shut down his storefront, so to speak, after his interactions with these women. That's how Jim Smith was born.

Matt C told me he tries to establish how well "they're going to be able to provide for a child financially first of all because I don't want a child to be born into a family that's struggling or bordering on destitute because they won't be able to have the things that they need." He also prefers to have a thorough conversation on the phone before meeting with potential candidates face-to-face. Once he and the recipient(s) are comfortable with one another he'll then work through the paperwork before going through with the donation process.

Christian and Juan selected their recipients based on a bigger picture idea as they insist on being known to the children from birth. "It was more about meeting and having the click with couples for us to want to donate to them. We wanted to ensure that the people we selected were going to be able to care for the baby, speak the same language about life, that we had some connections and similarities." They see what they are doing as a way to extend their family, so they are very fussy about who they choose to become part of their inner circle and donamily (donor family).

They selected five people for each of them to donate to as that seemed, what Juan says "manageable". They both prefer to only donate to same-sex or hetero couples due to the implications that are associated with donating to single women. As Christian told me, "Because once the baby is born they could potentially put your name on the birth certificate, and then you would be compelled to pay compensation and stuff like that. Whereas, if you just donate to lesbian couples or heterosexual couples you are likely covered. Because you can prove that it's a couple that you are helping through proof of FB, WhatsApp conversations etc. We felt more protected." They have a point and it's one I delve into a little later.

JLM generally doesn't discriminate at all with who he donates to bar one type. "I've donated to aboriginals; my daughter in Malta, her mother is half Maltese and half Greek. I don't discriminate on race, religion, ethnicity, whatever." He says "every woman who wants to have a child should be entitled to have a child. Because I am a Christian I step up to the plate and help out." While retired now, he saw it as his Christian duty, just as a committed lieutenant in the army. He's selflessly assisted families for decades both in a clinic, back in the days when LOTL (Lesbians on the Loose)—a monthly magazine—existed, and more recently through the Internet.

There is, however, one type of woman or couple he will not donate to. Ones that are adamant there will be no contact at all with the child.

"I don't contact any 'no contact women'. Some women want to totally screw their child from knowing their biological heritage. I don't agree with that, having lost so many children (through the clinic) so I don't reply to those women."

Thank goodness Chris is a genetics nerd. He didn't reveal to me how many families he was open to assisting, but he told me he doesn't "jeopardise the gene pool in any way. Hence, I'm careful in choosing recipient families in different cities and towns."

It was refreshing to learn that for the most part, these men cared where their sperm went. Just because a man chooses to be a donor doesn't mean he'll hand over his precious jiz to anyone. When I first set off on this path, I was unaware of this. I soon learned there are many men out there who have a specific type of woman or couple they choose to assist. Or at the very least, they have set their own standards.

> *"Riddle me, riddle me, randy ro*
> *My father gave me seeds to sow."*
> *- Ulysses, Greek hero*

A donee/recipient generally falls into these character profiles:

- Solo Roller - Straight, gay, transgender. Made a courageous decision to move forward solo despite circumstances. May or may not be reproductively aware.

- Flakes - Inconsistent messages - rude! Outlandish requests. Usually self-absorbed and disrespectful towards donors.

- Fill Me Up - Just as a puppy fills the heart, so too can a baby.

- Middle Aged Distressed - Run to the tick of the biological clock. Stressed, Anxious. Emotional. Time-oriented. Possibly Tindering for donors too.

- Man Haters - Women who loathe needing men for something. Anything!

- Guarded - Distrusting, stressed, tend to be hiding something about themselves.

- Early Starters - A generation ago they were in their prime to become mothers. Now they're considered young. Typically women under 25 who are bursting at the seams to become mothers.

- FOMO's (Fear of Missing Out) - I want one too! Suffers from baby envy.

- General Gay Couple - Relaxed, cool, easy to work with.

- Family Extender - Let's add another one. And another one. Obsessed with having lots of children. May have three kids and three different donor situations or former relationships. It's likely they receive Government childcare benefits.

- Family Completer - Women who've perhaps divorced or separated and would like a sibling for their only child/or children.

- Lesbian Links - When the ladies split and meet new partners they want another child together. Potentially link three or four families through children.

- Infertile Hetero Couple - Need assistance from a donor due to infertility.

- Plan A and SMC (single mothers by choice) - Mainly spinsters who rarely if ever had a relationship in their lives or those who would prefer to avoid relationships altogether to create a family.

- Transgender Couple - Need assistance from a donor due to the inability to reproduce together.

Like my chosen donor, I was a combination of a couple of "types".

Obviously middle-aged distressed and even a little FOMO. Yep, when I was with Ian a few of my friends were up the duff and I so wanted to move along this path at the same time with them. Seeing their bellies grow on their social media and then posts of their gorgeous bundles once they had arrived added to the frustrations of my 'never gonna happen' relationship.

This turned the volume up another couple of notches on the never-ending hand turning on that damn clickity, click bio clock.

While paying for sperm is a no-no for recipients, picking up out of pocket expenses is not only kindly accepted, it's advised to do so. SDA Adam has personally racked up some solid but conservative digits himself-his speedometer included! He used to spend a couple of hours in his car driving to and from recips homes to make donations but once he realised how much of his day he lost, and how it took away time from his family, he quickly changed how he operated.

Now recips travel to a selected spot that's more convenient for him.

After all, as far as he's concerned, he's the one giving out free baby juice and anyone who wants it sure as hell better make some effort to secure some. Donors can find it very telling when folks aren't willing to stretch themselves when it comes to helping themselves out with donations.

Fortunately, Adam has noticed a massive shift in these behaviours and attitudes within his circle here in Australia over the past couple of years.

# PART III

*MY BODY FELT ROUNDER THAN* usual. Soft. More voluptuous and feminine. I could feel it expanding as I sat there leaning up against the window staring at the clouds. I literally inhaled the teeny, tiny packet of pretzel and nuts that the stewardess handed me and sculled a cup of sauvignon blanc. Neither touched my expanding sides. My body was abuzz with fertile thoughts and my blood was gushing from head to toe. Every hair on my body was upright including my freshly manicured Tassie map. As we landed I was humming to a whole new Hokey Pokey melody.

*Chapter 15*

# Needles and Haystacks

*"A woman can never have too many lipstick options!"*
*— author unknown*

WHEN I FIRST FOUND MY way into what seemed like a wacky world, I had to understand the lingo and abbreviations. There sure was a stack of it but I learned fast just by reading different forums on the web. Any which way you choose to go about it, this is the unregulated way for producing children involving strangers that excludes relationship expectations.

ART (Assisted Reproductive Treatment) - Stands for any treatment procedures through a clinic, IUI (AI) using known sperm, IUI using donor sperm, IVF or ICSI.

AI is, of course, a popular fertility method used by women to conceive a child through sperm donation carried out at a fertility clinic.

The frozen sperm specimens have been screened for hereditary and genetic disorders and any serious diseases. These specimens may be donations from local donors or from other donors who have donated to cryobanks around the world.

Some known donors will only use a clinic to assist single women as it acts as a legal safety net. Some women may prefer this option too but both donor and recipient may have to jump through clinic hoops before the insemination can take place.

AI/or (HI) Home insemination using shipped clinic frozen sperm - When the tadpoles have been iced, they need to be thawed and then washed to eliminate any bad or slow-moving sperm; so that what's left is of optimum quality. It is then put into the recipient's womb using a syringe (bun gun) and sometimes with a catheter, although I don't recommend that without a doctor supervising. It's not a bad way to receive your can of sardines.

AI/HI (Home Insemination or Artificial Insemination) using fresh, sperm - involves the donor producing the donation into a sterile jar, handing it over to the recipient and then do what we Aussies say - 'the Harry Holt'. To the rest of the world it means 'to bolt'. The recipient then allows the semen to become viscous by warming the jar with body heat. Basically, it needs any lumps to liquefy into a smooth consistency but not become watery. Keeping it under an armpit or in a bra for approximately 30 minutes works great.

A woman can then inseminate herself (or partner) using a 5 or 10mL sterile syringe. Just to be clear, size does not matter here! A speculum may be used to ensure the syringe finds the right spot too. And there need not be any sexual contact or silly business with the donor at all.

Used to a lesser degree in HI/AI, are two other alternative conception devices. One requires using only a cervical cap opposed to a cup and syringe, and the other is a rather posh and much more refined technical instrument that takes that up a notch called, quite fittingly, The Stork OTC.

Cervical caps or soft caps are generally used to prevent making babies but they can also be used to assist in the very same thing they are protecting you from. They're usually used as a "barrier" method of birth control, because they're designed to block sperm from reaching the woman's egg. However, the opposite can be done to support sperm getting to the egg. You can either have the donor ejaculate directly into it, or you can transfer it from another clean container using a medical needleless syringe. Once the sperm is inside the cap you just insert it into your vagina as it will fit over your cervix. Then the swimmers are left to tube the wild rapids all the way to the ovum.

The Stork contraption takes the fuss out of handling semen and transferring it from cup to syringe to recipient. It has two main parts that assist in capturing the semen from the donor: the conceptacle and an applicator. The conceptacle part of the contraption consists of a cervical cap or soft cap which is the same type of "condom-like" sheath made out of silicone. Once the semen is collected, the sheath rolls off and is placed onto the tip of the applicator. The applicator is then used to insert the cap full of semen into the vagina and up to the opening of the cervix.

Then just as it is for cervical and soft caps, it's cuppa tea time. Or cleaning time. Movie time. Or whatever time. The cap can remain inside the cervix for a few hours so it's up to you what you do while you're hopefully whipping up a baby. The cap is removed just like a tampon with a string. Oh it's so sexy being a woman!

AI+ – This one I was not familiar with. Apparently the recipient is expected to help the donor produce the donation. I'm assuming with a little rub a dub, dub action.

Any of these AI methods are not only tried and proven ways to succeed in pregnancy, they are perhaps the best choices for putting some emotional distance between recipient and donor especially if they are friends or former lovers. These are the only procedures that may protect single women legally—maybe!

PI (Partial Insemination/Penetrative Insemination) – where the donor masturbates to the point of ejaculation and then inserts his penis into the recipient's vagina just prior to releasing the semen. There is minimal physical contact and intimacy, i.e. there is no kissing, oral sex, and exposure of or fondling of donee's breasts. It's what many men think of as 'sex without all the fun'. However, in light of that, it may offer a higher success rate to that of AI. It does pose some risk as it can take a few goes to get right, which can be not only frustrating for donee's, but costly in terms of time. To have gone through all the hoops only to have the donor fumble, lose his cool too soon or have insertion issues would be a monumental fail. To be blunt, a fuck up. A desperate geriatric can't have this happen EVER!

Adam bans promoting this method in his FB group because "it used to attract men with fetishes and a lot of these people we had issues with." He also says a lot of women have also experienced extreme discomfort with this method.

NI (Natural Insemination) - Good Ol' Fashioned S.E.X. - Rolling around in a haystack. It's the only natural form of procreation. Many guys prefer to do this for obvious reasons. And heck why not, after all it was the original baby-making way. Unfortunately, like slugging on a condom, single women don't have any protection with NI. This is because you're single. For the geriatrics, you're socially infertile remember?! Aka a social outcast! You get my point. As there isn't a second parent, the donor will be considered the father of the child. If you're in a partnership there is a chance, the donor might be considered the father of your child.

Natural insemination for women may fall under the highly stigmatised hammer just as one-night stands are. Some people might consider it dirty and salacious, but when you're doing it to make a baby, it isn't like that at all. There are many ways you can go about NI. It's up to you. But to get your head around pregnancy sex, well, it's generally not sexy at all. Just ask all the husbands and partners out there! It's a different type of sex with a person to create an outcome of creating a human being. It, like PI, is may not the least bit intimate and is often devoid of touch and kissing. Men who have abstained for a few days prior to this type of donation usually don't last long either.

On the other hand, some donors and donee's like to take an adventurous approach to NI and make it super fun for both parties. Heck, why not right? It could be the last time you have sex for a while and a 'make a baby' romp can be a truly magical experience with someone who only wants to gift you the ultimate win: the title of 'mother' and the pitter-patter of tiny feet.

John Cady is a NI only donor who runs a NI FB Group out of Houston, Texas. He's 45 years old, has a master's degree in engineering and works for a major oil company. He's donated to about twenty-five women and has twenty healthy children out of those donations. He even co-parents his fifteen-year-old daughter with the first woman he ever donated to, but they don't live together.

He says many women choose to do NI and other women would be perhaps surprised by that. "I've been told by many women that they prefer the conception of their baby to be the natural way, and furthermore, they simply enjoy sex and want to make the most of it. Sex is a pleasurable activity for both men and women, so why try and pretend it's not?"

Even though this is his preferred method of donating, he says, "If a woman thinks it's horrible to use that method, and if that is what they believe, then I will never attempt to talk them into using NI." But this is the only method he uses. He's had women get angry at him for refusing to change his method telling him that if he truly cared about women he'd help them by any means possible. "Well, that's fine for them to say that but they don't know my heart. I truly want to help women have a much-wanted baby, but it has to be NI. If they get angry over my stance then I wish them all the luck in the world in finding the donor they want. It just won't be me. I can't be guilt-tripped into helping someone like that."

"I understand why there is such bitterness from some women over men who use NI as the donation method. I think the real issue is those donors that advertise using AI, and then when they have the women interested or on the hook suddenly change their mind and insist upon NI.

This is holding the woman hostage as the donor will often wait until she is near ovulation and hopes she will be so desperate for a baby that she will agree to the use of intercourse as the donation method rather than the agreed upon AI. For those so-called donors that do this, I hope you are offended when I say you are just about the lowest of scum possible."

John has met with single and married couples to perform what may be a new term for insemination: XI, which stands for erotic or exotic insemination. "We would meet and basically treat it like a mini-vacation where I'd be available to go out for dinner, maybe have some non-sexual fun, and then have sex two or three times a day in-between our activities."

"It tended to make things more like a dating situation for the single women rather than a clinical sexual encounter. It gave them a brief connection with me so when they conceived their baby they could think of the two or three day event as something they enjoyed doing. Once, a married couple was much the same as I was invited to their home in a beautiful part of the country and for a few days we relaxed, they took me site seeing into the mountains, and had plenty of good food...and of course sex three times a day (literally morning, noon, and night)."

From John's perspective, he didn't think of this as anything "but a good time with potential friends that had a happy ending when she got pregnant and later delivered a healthy son" (the husband had a condition where he didn't produce sperm).

He told me about another married woman who went on a vacation to Europe by herself to cavort with a donor with her husband's blessing.

She went sightseeing, dined out and enjoyed her solo time. Then, when she was in her prime ovu window she met with her donor. They enjoyed some good sex over a couple of days, then she flew home to her husband with a positive result. Another story John shared was about a couple who had their donor live with them until she got pregnant!

As John says, "If you are going to do the deed with a stranger to get pregnant there is no rule that you can't make the most of it and enjoy yourself. I'm not saying you have to go on a vacation, but the dirty little secret is that it generally feels good when a penis enters a vagina, so why pretend it doesn't? Make the most of it."

*Chapter 16*

# CONtroversy

*"A shady business never yields a sunny life."*
*- B. C. Forbes, journalist*

ANNIE, A LONG TIME HOPEFUL donee in Perth, got the run around by a few donors she believes were never able to impregnate her. Determined to have a third child, she found herself carelessly settling for semen from donors whom she says were "shady and sterile men."

She and I connected through the SDA group of which she had been a member of for a couple of years trying to add to her clan. She told me she felt vulnerable to the whole process but pushed forward despite all the red flags of con artists. The urgency to conceive was stressful and she made sure every month, no matter what, she would try with a private donor. Unfortunately, her desperation outweighed logic and therefore came at a cost of her choosing wisely.

Her quest to land another baby outside a clinic had her pay for monthly membership on a couple of donor sites, join online Facebook groups and also sign up on the Just A Baby app. Although consistently trying month after month over years, she said she had no luck in any of these arenas.

As a middle-aged woman, she then started to question donors who weren't having success with her or anybody else. And when the requests from donors were specifically for NI not AI, she got disenchanted by this whole process. She said, "you only have to look at Adam Hooper's massive success only doing AI and you have to question their motives."

As a married man with 2 children, Adam only ever donates using a cup and syringe. He's been able to assist a bunch of women over the years using the straightforward HI method. He's above board and expects everyone in his FB group to operate with the same good intentions too. Despite the dodgy behaviour of the odd one or two peeps, he's adamant that this route is by far a better one than IVF. He believes fresh sperm offered from a private donor is by far superior to that of frozen stuff bought from a clinic. As he said in our interview on ABC's 7.30 news show "fresh is best". This one-liner still totally cracks me up but his point is a valid one as he has a bunch of babies to prove it.

Annie told me she moved through four men, who she believes had motives that were not completely altruistic. The first few men she hooked up with either wanted financial compensation or pushed for NI when they were actually infertile. She tried five natural cycles with one guy who according to her "was not easy as he was 'very introverted and basically impotent.'" He was appealing to her because he could donate daily, which for a mid 40s woman was essential. "He was a single guy and could do five days in a row. I could say to him 'I am very regular I am going to be needing you on these days' and he'd be available."

By the last insemination, she felt like something wasn't right. She finally asked him to produce his semen results which he eventually did after another cycle. As she looked the paperwork over, her gut twisted and tightened. She felt the numbers before her eyes had been doctored which only supported her suspicions that he wasn't as fertile as he had proclaimed. She figured he was most likely just in it for the sex and was, therefore, wasting her time.

Another donor she reconnected with after a brief break told her that he was offered cash to assist other women who were willing to pay him for his service. He was testing her to see if she'd chime in and make a bid. Annie knew this wasn't good practice or ethical but what could she do? Pay to play or lose her chance that cycle? She didn't capitulate, so of course, his sperm went to the highest bidder. With hot flushes now upon her, it's fair to say she got monumentally screwed over.

However, I dare say, it's easy to blame and throw shade on the shitty donor than be rational and take some responsibility for one's own bad choices too. Irrelevant of the donors' behaviours, Annie ultimately screwed herself out of a baby by screwing around with jerks.

John Cady who only donates via NI agrees that there are a random few out there who don't donate sperm in good faith. Private donors may tell women they must do NI or they won't get their sperm which forces women into a corner when they're ovulating. "Yes, there are some very underhanded donors out there who prey on vulnerable women hoping to get the chance to change their minds once they agree to AI."

While his FB group is for those who only do NI, even JC is disgusted with men who bring that kind of murkiness into his group. His advice is to stay firm on your principles, "never give in; just go elsewhere. If you go through with it you will hate yourself for the rest of your life for compromising your principles with a true scumbag." My thoughts here - think about the child! You're hoping to bring a beautiful, pure little being into the world who shouldn't be created in or around vulgar or low vibrational energy!

Some donors absolutely believe that NI is more concise than AI and that's why they push for it especially when recips are over 40. The more the sperm is "man-handled", the less likely it is to survive. Eliminating the plastic cups and silicone caps means it's not only not exposed to environment elements that may alter its quality, it also lessens the risk of human error. There's no known research whether one works better over the other, only success stories from women willing to share their stories.

Another recipient who contacted me via Facebook told me that her potential private benefactor donor who was married with 3 kids and pregnant with their forth, only donates after having sex with his wife.

"He said that the way they do it is that they have sex and then he orgasms into a cup or whatever." She added "they want to shag to give me the donation and in order to do that, they are only available at night...I thought what a pain in the ass."

This may or may not be considered shady behaviour due to our differing personal views and opinions, but this one had me scratching my head. Mainly because I didn't value the donor's actions as being entirely altruistic.

Other devious behaviours include but are not limited to; deliberate donor no-shows since there's so much riding on those peak days, distasteful 'public-gutter' and social media chat, married men secretly donating, sharing images of donor children without consent and knowingly spreading STI's.

Interestingly, the community is pretty tight, even across oceans, so the odd character who is more shoddy than virtuous will get outed then hastily booted from donor circles.

Apart from the firefighter whom I extinguished in one conversation when he tried to get some hot n sexy banter from me, I didn't have any issues with shady dudes. I guess it's because my approach was professional, responsible and well informed. I was serious about my outcome and couldn't afford to throw away valuable time on someone who could be considered a con-artist.

*Chapter 17*

# The Deed

*"Instead of worrying about what you cannot control, shift your energy to what you can create." -*
*Roy T. Bennett, The Light in the Heart*

YES, I WAS NERVOUS. MOSTLY excited. And completely relieved. I wasn't sure if this was going to work. Just doing it though made me feel like a weight had been taken off my shoulders and I was with someone who got it, who cared. He made it his personal mission, too, and truly wanted success for me.

I frantically looked for signage directing me to the shuttle pick up location once I'd landed, but I was distracted by my phone's incoming texts. It was blowing up from The DSS Crusade Committee who wanted to ensure I had landed safely and to let me know they were excited and also freaking out, with me. We were all feeling a mish-mash of emotions, but I knew they were ridiculously curious to know what Mr Stork looked like in the flesh. After ten minutes of watching a few vans come and go, I called the hotel to find out where mine was. It pulled up a few minutes later and I hopped on.

I had more time to speculate and think up some silly scenarios of what was just ahead of me. I texted him to find out how far away he was. He was only twenty minutes from arriving, which meant I wouldn't have long to check in and wash away some of the nervous energy under a hot running shower.

I made sure I was the first one to jump out of the bus and wait at reception. Having no luggage was a massive plus for allowing me to rush about. I grabbed my hotel key and hot-footed it straight to the elevator. I wasn't sure if Mr Stork had beaten me there and was sitting in the bar opposite the foyer. The bar was bustling with people and I hoped he didn't see me before I managed to at least put some makeup on. I know I wasn't there to impress him. I know it wasn't a date. Still, I couldn't have handled him rejecting me saying I wasn't worthy of his goods.

I was only in the room for about five minutes when he texted me to let me know he was in the bar area. I so needed a drink; I told him I'd meet him down there. I jumped in the shower, did a quick last minute body hair check, cleaned my teeth, spritzed some body mist all over me and made my way down to the lobby bar. I texted him and as I approached he turned around. I felt an immediate rush of fear, so said I'd grab us some drinks from the bar. I was bummed when he only asked for a mineral water as this was one of those times that alcohol and adrenalin were a perfect mix.

I waited to be served just out of his view behind a pillar at the bar. I figured this was my only chance to call one of my wing women to get some reassurance to stay or flee. I reached into my bag, grabbed my phone and dialled Kim. I told her I was flipping out and didn't think I could go through with it. She reminded me that my hormones would be doing backflips right about now and just take a moment to assess the situation more clearly.

She was right. I ordered two glasses of house wine. One to throw down right that second at the bar and another to take over and sip a little more civilised-like with Mr Stork while he drank his mineral water. My head was spinning. It was all so full on. We hadn't hung out in the flesh before and now I wasn't sure if we had rushed things. I hadn't experienced anything like this before. I was moving straight to the punch line without downing some punch, or something with a kick first.

We went up to the room. I thought I was flipping out before but now I was seriously freaking out. I couldn't believe I was there; that it was real. I was meeting with a complete stranger to attempt making a baby. He had really shown up. He was real. This was happening. All of my work to make something happen had gotten me here... in this hote room.

I told him I needed some time to take it all in. And I needed another drink. I shuffled back down to the bar and ordered another glass of wine. Two down and another being sunk as I travelled back up to level six. Or as the Kiwi's say sux or sex...oh, and there it now was. The 3 letter word was clearly at the forefront of my mind.

A combination of wine, adrenaline and elation had me buzzing. Not to forget my hormones that had literally added an extra inch to my waistline just thinking about becoming pregnant. My body was ready, it wanted this but my head needed an extra moment. We had been chatting now for a couple of hours and I'd finally began to relax. I felt comfortable for us to move forward with the insemination.

He leaned into his bag very furtively and pulled out a syringe. I looked over both shoulders and noticed the blinds behind the curtains were slightly ajar. I jumped up to fix them as I was sure we had eyeballs on us from somewhere. This had me feeling like we were about to engage in a shonky shoot up session. I noticed I'd been holding my breath. Next, he revealed the sterile cup. Phew. He was here for the right reasons. I exhaled.

It was now quite late and finally it felt right to give it a go. I climbed into bed. Mr Stork hopped to the bathroom. My blood was gushing from my head to the toes. My body wanted to be impregnated. It was like my egg was waiting on the widow's lookout for her lucky swimmer to appear, entice and completely ravish him. My body was aching for a baby.

It was perhaps five minutes and Mr Stork had done what he came here to do. He handed me his 'bun gun' which was loaded with hope. I lined the swimmers up on the starting block, then once that whistle blew, out they sprung onto the winding course. The race upstream was officially underway. I then turned toward the bed head and pulled out my best Viparita Karani yet. This is a yoga term for being upside down.

I'd kept this one in my back pocket. Now was time to pull out guidance from a higher self. Fingers crossed and legs waving in the air just wasn't going to cut it.

My mind moved energy in downward waves swooshing it all around my pelvis. I prayed for just one to have the smarts to follow these strong electrical pulses and was limber enough to navigate my tightly knotted body's 'non yoga-ish' innards. At the very least, I needed those bad boys to have some serious FOMO.

Half an hour later, Mr Stork fired off another wad of swimmers. Repeat Viparita Karani. Although this time a little less knotted. I am sure the blood rush to the head was intensified with the wine. While I lay there, the mind chatter began pondering the realisation that our domance had just escalated to official donorship status.

I also hoped Ms. Mew Kus hadn't sent down a resolute line of defence. I needed every competing swimmer to wipe out any obstacles in their way. The more taddies, the more chances. This was one of those times where I was on board with the 'everybody gets a trophy' mentality.

I reminded myself to stay on the offensive and tap positive baby juju thoughts, fuel them with affirmations and to consider myself pregnant now. After all, my body (perhaps still just my mind) had seemingly taken that voluptuous approach already.

By this time we were starving and before the kitchen closed I ordered us room service. Mr Stork re-energised on steak. I devoured more fish. Any uneasiness that existed in the beginning had completely evaporated. We were just two mates hanging out like we had done so over the internet. Our pillow talk had taken us to 3am before we realised, and then we passed out for a few hours. When I awoke, Mr Stork had another round to offload. He handed me a barrel full of fresh swimmers.

Room service was on their game today. I gladly accepted his kind offer and launched them as far into my uterus as they could go before breakfast.

We then both scurried out of the room and made our way down to the airport shuttle bus. It was still early and I had a couple of hours to kill before my flight, so I grabbed us some scrambled eggs before paying for his ride back to the city and we went our separate ways.

It was like, "Thanks for coming!" Only it was, "REALLY thanks for coming..." It was the first time I could say that and wholly mean it.

On my flight home, I calculated the estimated investment I had made thus far:

Total expenditure (in %)

- Emotional: 5 per cent
- Mental: 80 per cent - Started high and then went down to about 25 per cent. Hardest part was counting my days and being sure I was 100 per cent in my fertile window
- Spiritual: 0

- Financial: Flights, dinner, breakfast, hotel room, bus ticket, bar drinks, AI kit, taxi home. Half the cost of one IUI using international donor sperm specimen at a clinic (Way less for those who don't need to travel)
- Ovu cycles: 0 wasted. Successful first round.

*Fear and sweat percentage inconclusive

The IUIs I had at the fertility clinic only had up to 0.5 mL of semen, but my known donor was able to supply me with approximately 23 mL in 3 deliveries. That would be the same as 46 vials worth of clinic semen excluding any type of cryoprotectant.

That's over AU$11,000 in value to minimally purchase local Aussie semen if his was segregated in individual vials under WHO guidelines. Then, approximately another AU$49,680 to have it injected by a doctor.

If I was to purchase international semen of the same quantity the cost would be AU$55,200 and about another fifty thousand to have that inseminated by the doc.

Now, of course, I wouldn't ever do that many IUIs but I've just shared this comparison so you get the jizz, er hm, gist. With sperm quality and quantity of that calibre there's really no need to do NI unless you want to. The likelihood of pregnancy isn't just possible, it's highly probable especially if you haven't had any fertility issues. Now let's look at the other numbers...the ones that truly matter.

My donor had a sperm count of over a billion but have rounded down (to keep it real) to 800 million per 10mL with 66 per cent progressive motility.

10mL x 800 million+ x 66 per cent progressive motility

Compared with a WHO qualified specimen from a clinic:

0.5mL x 39 million x 32 per cent progressive motility (of course, these are estimates because I wasn't told the real figures)

Combined with my total costs for my private donor sperm - a few hundred dollars on flights, hotel, meals, transport for both of us as well as OPKs. All up, I spent about half what I did on one IUI.

Other out of pocket expenses for my entire two year 'make me a mother' crusade (which includes my IUI attempts) such as vitamins, acupuncture, dentist, naturopath visits, etc. brings my financial cost up to at least another thousand or so. However, these costs can also be considered as overall general health and wellness outlay. It's crazy to think that every day, or every other day, everyday men stand under a hot shower releasing that stuff down the drain. So the value of it ultimately depends on how much you place on its means to an end.

Thinking about it makes me want to break out and sing Monty Python's little satirical musical number, 'Every Sperm Is Sacred' performed in their film 'The Meaning of Life'. It's a hysterical piss-take of Catholicism which forbids making babies through artificial means.

In the skit, Michael Palin plays a poor Catholic father who must sell his 63 children for medical experimentation as he and his wife (played by the late Terry Jones) can no longer afford to take care of and provide for them.

Their kids question them as to why they don't just practice contraception which would seemingly be a no-brainer easy solution. Their father responds by explaining to them that it's against God's wishes to do so.

They then break out into song.

It inspired me to tap my creativity and piece one together too:

*Every sperm is desired*
*Every sperm is hired*
*Every sperm is a little person*
*No need to buy em*
*Hit up a known donor for em*
*Every sperm is a worm*
*Every sperm needs a turn*
*Every sperm could be an Olympic swimmer*
*It's their chance to be a winner*
*Okay...my lyrics aren't really comparable to the prose masters.*

*However, it did provide me with many hours of amusement that I could apparently afford to throw down the loo.*

# Chapter 18
# Time Bending Tips

*"And sure enough, even waiting will end...*
*if you can just wait long enough."*
*- William Faulkner, American writer*

*"Have but a little patience, a week's patience, and it shall be."*
*- IV, Scythrop's Fate*

SO, OF COURSE, THE GREAT question re-emerges: what do you do for the following two weeks while you wait to find out if it worked? You could take the steps to start writing your memoir like I did—then figure out a path for all your written words like I have done. As it turned out for me, I couldn't wait to share what I had learned during my pregnancy crusade. It became my focus regardless of what the pending pregnancy result would be. I also had convinced myself that it could take months for it to happen, so I had mentally prepared my BFP to be a negative read.

While I don't have answers on how to speed up inertia, I can offer some creative ways to origami these painstakingly slow hours to make them feel as though they're actually forcing the hands of the clock forward.

Some of my tips for bending time:

- Get certified in first aid. Completing a course to accrue some lifesaving skills may not just be helpful for yourself and your future little one(s) but also for any situation you might find yourself where others need assistance. Without a doubt my top 2WW distraction!

- Research and write your birth plan - If you're anything like me, you will be clueless about this. I was fixated on just staying pregnant and didn't focus on the end result until I needed to. Which was basically when I was lying in my bed in the hospital. My birth plan was to have no birth plan. Roll with it.

In hindsight, it would have been nice to understand what was ahead so I was educated and could make informed decisions on the birth and what life would be like thereafter. It didn't mean I became obsessive about I wanted to have happen, it just meant I was aware of the options available to me. For instance, I didn't know that I needed to organise an umbilical cord plan for cord blood banking before I went to the hospital. I thought I could organise that from my hospital bed up until I had been induced. A kit takes one to three business days to get to you so if you want to store your cord for stem cells, this is something you'll want to have organised.

- Take a trip out of town - A change of scenery can speed up time. Well, not exactly, unless you head to a time zone ahead of the one you're in. New sights can break up the monotony of being in your everyday environment and get you out of your head. Spend some time with your besties, hang out in some cute little cafes, trek through forests you've never walked through or feel the sand between your toes along beaches and coastlines you've never visited.

- Fill up your dance card! If you're single, go on some dates. Heck, why not? If you're up the duff you may not get any horizontal action with another human for at least a year. Besides, you don't know if you're pregnant or not. But what's it matter anyway, you're still single right? My friend Pim told me a story about going on a date with a woman who had only recently become pregnant. She'd told him she'd had "a little procedure" done since they had last seen one another. It confused him at first as he really didn't know what to do with that information and what that meant for him and her. What it did do, was paint a picture of what was ahead if he was interested in travelling down that same road holding her hand.

This is a situation that will no doubt become more common as more and more single women go and take care of 'it' themselves. I just think go for it. You may meet the one you've been searching for, realise your date is a good work contact or may even be someone to catch up with every now and then. If things take off with a special one then he'll either hang about and jump in with both feet (bonus) or bolt faster than lightning. If he's a single guy this could be a way to fast track him to parenthood. Either way, you win. Dinner, a night out, distraction, another story to tell when you're 90 years old.

• Stream a TV series - An obvious one I know. But if there's any time to lose yourself in an entire season or several this is it. Take your mind off yourself and obsess over the lives of others. Never will Netflix be your daily obsession in such a good way till now!

So create a favourites list and get binging. These long indulgent couch potato days will soon be a distant memory so stock up on all those shows you've been putting on hold until now. Trust me on this one, in an instant your box will only be blaring out "Dora; The Explorer", "The Wiggles" or "Play School". Oh, and on repeat too ;)

• Kon Mari your wardrobe - Make way for some maternity and new mum wear! Clear out all the clothes that you haven't fit into for at least a year and pop in one pile. Create another pile of clothes that could work as maternity wear; and also separate your winter and summer clothes that you DO wear. Box up whichever season you won't need for the following six months. Anything with holes in it, is completely worn or dishevelled needs to go into another pile. Choose one or two items from this pile if you think you'll wear them in the garden, painting or doing any house renovations. The rest need to be cut into rags or tossed.

Make another pile of clothes that you love but NEVER wear. This could be your special occasion outfits, former bridesmaid dresses, sentimental pieces or designer bargains you picked up but still have no place to wear. From the 'too small', fancy clothes, winter and summer piles that you don't wear, pop into a bag or hang on a rack—it's time to turn your old clothes into baby clothes cash! Take pictures of each item and post on Ebay, FB or book a spot to set up a stall at your local markets.

- Create a story book - A treasured item for your child! You can put loads of time and effort into personally crafting a family ancestry scrapbook, life book or story book for your little one when they arrive. This is a great way to incorporate your child's unique conception story into their night-time storytelling so they'll always know the lay of the land of who they are and how they came to be. From ordering paper to colouring in a family tree, this creative project will suck up the hours and have you forgetting you took on this craft project purely to distract yourself. Without a doubt, it'll be a treasured item that your child will be thankful for in years to come. Look online for inspiration on Pinterest or hit up Etsy.

- Plant a tree - Yes, why not grow something while you're on your own 'planting a seed' mission? Pop a seed into the earth and get your hands elbow deep in rich, fertile soil as you smother a tiny kernel over with Mother Nature's finest blend of nurturing plant organics. This is not only pure earth erotica, it deeply connects you with source, mothership's intoxicating fuel for life.

- Acquire skills - Maybe you want to arm yourself with the know how to snap great photos of your soon to be here newborn by taking a photography course. Perhaps you want to upskill for when you go back to work after you've completed your maternity leave. Or you're pondering accumulating a whole set of new skills so you can create a life that gives you more time at home with your baby. Or you may just want to become more tech savvy on your computer by learning short cuts, programs and software that you just haven't had a chance to conquer....UNTIL NOW!

Udemy, among many others, have a stack of digital courses which will surely both entertain and inform you. There is probably a course for anything you can think up. Most courses can be started at any time so can be worked in to suit your cycles and waiting periods, which hopefully doesn't end up as a physical period.

- Get creative  - Blend smelly potions together to make a bunch of eco soaps, bath salts and candles. Not only will these come in handy for spoiling yourself when you're pregnant but they make great 'feel goods' once you bring bubs home. There are a bunch of how-to videos on YouTube and articles online sharing info on how you can make your own self-care products. From buying a few soap moulds to buying salt in bulk, making luscious eco-friendly and baby sensitive products won't break the bank and doesn't require a science degree.

- Clear out your storage area; Clear out some space - This is one of the best tasks you could set yourself to do. Sheds, garages, dens, storerooms and spare bedrooms are all places we tend to put things when we're either rushed, can't think of what to do with something or think we'll just hide it so it's out of the way.

Over the years you accumulate a bunch more stuff and before you know this chunk of real estate is a resting place to a bunch of random items. So get in there and give them a good wipe over then take a snap and advertise them on FB marketplace, eBay, Craigslist, Gumtree, in your local newspaper or on your local community board. It's time to turn your stuff into cash so you can buy that sassy (second-hand) stroller or go on that babymoon.

- Make a date night phone list and get dialling - Call a different friend or family member a night and catch up with them! We all get caught up in our worlds and especially so when we're on a baby-making mission. This tunnel vision can have us neglect our wider group of friends and family. So, for the next 13 nights, check in with old high school pals, neighbours, college friends and extended family members to say g'day.

- Do a two week yoga challenge - Many yoga and meditation studios, and even gyms, offer free trial days or weeks. So, sign up for a class a day. Not only do you just have to show up, but you'll be supporting your physical, mental and emotional health as well as being surrounded by a bunch of people who you can potentially connect with or at the very least, offer some conversation to distract you from getting in your head.

- Get reading - Buy two or three books and set yourself the challenge to get through them by diving in every night and all weekend! Hit your local second-hand book store or jump on Amazon and buy some inspiring new releases or perhaps you've promised yourself that one day you'll read the entire 'Harry Potter' or 'Lord of the Rings' series. Well, your 2WW is the perfect time to lose yourself in these phenomenal stories.

- Tour your area - You don't have to get on a plane or drive for miles to cut ties with your everyday life and embark on a path of revitalisation. It's just a shift in perspective, but all of a sudden there are new sights, smells, tastes and sounds right outside your doorstep. This cycle is the cycle for hometown tourism aka 'la budget touriste'. It's also the perfect solution for satisfying a travel itch (if you have one), learn more about what exists beyond your backyard and shake up the monotony without, drum roll please, draining the wallet. Being a local tourist isn't always about exploring new places, it can also be about seeing old places in new ways.

- Teach yourself to knit - Why wait for gifts when you can knock your socks off by knitting your own blankies, hats and mittens?! They won't go astray when the little one comes.

- Tune out the ticking tock with some Transcendental (TM) or Vedic Meditation (VM). A group course of VM typically spans four days, for a couple of hours at a time. This is a superb way to shut the little voice in that head down for a while. Or, if by chance all the planets align, perhaps you could head to a Vipassana centre to drown out your thoughts with stillness?

- Volunteer - Use this time productively by deflecting that anxious energy from yourself by giving nurturing cuddles to an animal in need of loads of love. Many shelters would welcome extra hands on deck and the animals would be thrilled to have attention that would otherwise be wasted on stress.

*Chapter 19*
# My BFP ;)

*"Success is getting what you want, happiness is wanting what you get"*
*- author unknown*

*HAVING GONE THROUGH A FEW* two week waits, I felt I was an expert at getting through the hours with some kind of poise. I didn't clean out any garage, landscape the garden or immerse myself in every episode of "The Handmaid's Tale". My research and writing kept me completely engaged so I didn't feel a need to remind myself what day it was, keep a close eye on the hands of a clock or be dictated by what was happening in my knickers. I felt if anything, that the hours between 9am and 5pm went too fast and I couldn't get enough done in a day.

Yes. Writing this book, thankfully, had occupied me enough to have this 2WW fly by. Mr Stork contacted me on Day 16 to investigate if there was one lucky winner from the 'great anti-gravity' swim. Mrs. Menses had not shown up so I hadn't yet reported back to him. He was confident this was a positive sign; however, I didn't want to get my hopes up. My box felt like it was going to drop between my legs at any given moment.

I had two home pregnancy tests in my drawer and hadn't even considered using them until we chatted. As soon as I got off the phone, though, I decided to use one. I tottered off to the bathroom, peed on the stick and sat on the bowl staring at the flashing test. I really hadn't put much hope into this as I had been let down so many times before. I felt like I had racked up a bunch of failures over the past 18 months and this was just going to be another to add to the list.

While my thighs rested on the toilet seat and my limp, white cheeks dangled over the bowl of still water below, I replayed the conversation I'd had just a few days ago with Lucas. He had finally responded to my message as he was still keen to donate. After a few hours of getting to know one another over the phone, he had become my back up plan. Plan B. Finally I found a legit back up plan! We got along like a house on fire, which had me contemplate that perhaps he was a better donor choice.

He was only a two hour drive from me, which long term, made it more economically viable than travelling to Melbourne every few weeks.

After spacing out for a few minutes, my attention was brought back to the pee stick. It showed a BFN. I threw it in the bin, wrote to Mr Stork to let him know it didn't work and got on with my day. He seemed shocked by the result and continued to probe me to figure out how on earth it had failed.

I'd concluded that my cycle was just out of whack and I miscalculated my ovulation. With the two different reads on the OPK's and making moves on Day 14, it seemed, I needed to jump earlier. I didn't get bogged down in it. I had resigned myself that this was just one of the many bumps along the road to get me to the desired bump I would just have to get over. With many, many more cycles to come.

Five days later, I met with Chez for a much needed coffee break. She had already ordered for the both of us by the time I arrived, but before I pulled up a chair opposite her, I told her I felt Aunty Flo had just dropped in and I'd better handle it. I took off to the loo where I wasn't greeted by the river of red I was expecting. Instead, I was shocked to see a pool of white.

I relayed this information to Chez, who didn't flinch about the graphic detail I brought back to the table. She demanded I take another home pregnancy test of which I reiterated that I could feel my period was literally edging its way to say g'day. She informed me that's what pregnancy felt like. Once we finished our coffees, she dragged me down the road, purchased a kit and sent me off to the supermarkets "high end" public powder room.

To entertain her, I peed on the stick and then had her join me in the cubicle while we both eagle-eyed the flashing dots for what seemed like several minutes. Finally, after a couple of minutes the dots disappeared and in absolute jaw down shock, they were replaced with the word PREGNANT.

Twenty-one days after the deed, it was finally revealed that one speedy tadpole had indeed been the victor. We both looked at each other stunned. Holy shit, a BFP. Agape, we locked eyes. Hers sparkled back at me. She bellowed, "I knew it!" before we embraced, jumped up and down, then called my committee's third member, Kim, to share this insane news.

In that moment an immediate shift occurred. It was like in that very instant all my emotional distress and frustration evaporated. My skew-whiff solo strategy worked on my first attempt and now I was growing my very own Piscean, a baby Nemo. While there are a stack of cute baby bump nicknames like Bean and Peanut out there, mine for no reason at all, was promptly dubbed Widgetty Grub.

Later that night, with this positive news barely having a chance to seep in, DOUBT took the opportunity to trickle through. It had me second guessing the result. I wasn't convinced it was correct. After all, the one I'd taken only five days earlier had an alternative result.

Unconvinced, I visited a local GP a few days later to request a blood test. She advised me that home pregnancy tests were 99 per cent accurate and she didn't feel I needed one. I pushed for it. A few days later, I followed up with the doctor to get the blood test result. It was positive.

As time went on, though, there still wasn't any physical indication that I was up the duff. I didn't feel ill, tired, or turned off by food, which really confused me; so I wouldn't, couldn't, let myself believe. In fact, even though I had a positive home pregnancy test and doctor administered blood test, followed by a Harmony test (NIPT) at six weeks (which rules out some chromosomal abnormalities such as Down syndrome (trisomy 21), Edwards syndrome (trisomy 18) and Patau syndrome (trisomy 13), I waited until my first scan, to finally believe that I was actually carrying the beginnings of a wee bitty human. Until I saw that heart beating, I did not believe that this really and truly was really true.

I followed my higher self, which included a little of my gut and mind, gave up on IVF, navigated my own path and wholeheartedly believed in myself that I could do this. And I did.

It's a relief. It's joyous. It's gratitude. Yes, in the moment you see that '+ sign' on your pregnancy pee stick, hear the 'yes' from the doctor, or in my case, the faint heartbeat from the monitor, you just feel so incredibly grateful for the donor who has just made your dream come true. Nothing but immense gratitude.

It seemed as though my period was oscillating. I was braced for its arrival. Then, when nothing showed up, I remained sceptical. This was new territory and I still wasn't really sure how the early stages of pregnancy unfolded or any phase of pregnancy for that matter. I stalled sharing a pic of the positive pee stick with Mr Stork for another week as I didn't want to make the grand announcement only to have to retract it hours later. He was pretty hopeful and sure it had worked but wanted to start figuring out our insem plan for the following month. I stalled on making those arrangements so told him that while I didn't feel confident, I did have a positive result. He was thrilled telling me he had already shared my (his/ our) wonderful news with his mother!

Mr Stork: Oh you - Aunty Flo just didn't arrive. Ha! You were funny last night about your period.....oh just missed. Could still be coming. Very funny.

Hayley: Well, periods can be weird.

Mr Stork: Yeah

Hayley: And I've come to believe it's too crazy for me to have a kid! I'm gobsmacked it worked!

Mr Stork: Haha. You did say you were on a mission.

Hayley: Yes.

Mr Stork: I have to be honest my mum knows.

Hayley: That you got me up the duff?

Mr Stork: Yep....

Hayley: You tell her my sitch?

Mr Stork: 41. One go. Bam. She loves it.....i told her you were 41.... she said to me.....it's so great that you both met so you can become a mum.....and then in typical mum style she said she'd love to see a picture of the child.

A few days later, I cancelled all my specialist appointments, threw out my packet of Clomid and called Doc Merlin to let him know. I couldn't wait to tell him and the nurses I had conceived on my first fresh cycle without any intrusive tests, drugs or procedures. I also contacted Lucas to let him know his bowl of swimmers could be set free.

# PART IV

*"The public is a ferocious beast; one must either chain it or flee from it." – Voltaire, writer*

IF THERE IS ONE THING we humans have never seemed to evolve out of, it is public JUDGEMENT, which is one of the reasons I was 20 weeks along before I went public about my pregnancy. All the riff raff in the media had me buying into the high occurrence of late miscarriages or still births at my age.

I felt like this pregnancy thing was a lot like the board games Snakes and Ladders combined with Jenga. Every move, so delicate that it would directly impact or influence the other.

When SDA Adam informed me that a reporter from the ABC was keen to do a story on women skipping the clinics for this internet route. I decided to put my hand up and speak out. It wasn't an easy decision at first as, even though, I was writing a book about my journey, I wasn't planning on using my real name. I found being pregnant came with a huge dose of courage. I had my cool 'nom de plume' worked out, but while I was mid-way through the first draft it dawned on me that for my story to mean anything to anyone, it had to have a face.

I needed to attach me to my own story. I knew it wouldn't have the impact it needed or reach the people it was meant otherwise. It wasn't something I was planning to do, but I realised I would be hiding behind it—allowing SHAME and JUDGEMENT to have a hold over me. And I was damned if I'd give them that much power.

I wouldn't have had the guts to do the TV interview had I not decided to put my name on my book. Courage is funny that way, its momentum grew as I accepted and realised my place in the world.

For the most part, I was so relieved that I could shake off all the energy required for figuring out how the heck I was going to make a baby and now just focus on the next phase—staying pregnant and birthing a healthy bub. It was exhausting getting to this point and I just wanted to be present.

It was also time for me to share the news with my mother, who I hadn't yet said a peep to about this. I think her heart stopped beating while her ears bounced sound around trying to piece together my words.

To say she was surprised is a massive understatement. She never thought she'd ever be a grandmother in this lifetime.

The pregnancy was breezy and I feel guilty saying that as I know it's not like that for so many women. I didn't have one craving. I didn't suffer from morning sickness. I continued on my merry way, just living life. The last few weekends before I popped out my precious little human, I took it upon myself to indulge in some short getaways as a single woman to enjoy solo time, full conversations and sleep.

*Chapter 20*

# Child Free in the City

*"Families with babies and families without babies are sorry for each other."*
*- Ed Howe, novelist*

IT WAS JUST A FEW weeks before I was scheduled for my induction at the hospital, when I flew to Sydney to hang with my girlfriends, Bec and Jackie.

As I was nearing the end of my pregnancy, I was indulging in my last ever girls getaway as a "selfish" single woman. I hadn't really gone out over the past nine months so it was nice to make an effort and step out for the night. It was a luscious February afternoon and it seemed that all of the city's suits were out and about enjoying it, too. The three of us caught up at a swanky rooftop bar in Barangaroo where we could revel in the electric vibe.

Had we not been chatting about my pending labour, I could have easily forgotten I was sitting there in maternity wear. Both mothers, the girls knew exactly what was ahead of me. It was the one part of this journey that did not excite me. Still, they promised me I would survive just as they did and assured me that I've 'got this'.

The following day, I organised a late afternoon catch up with a couple of other girlfriends by Luna Park. Both were friendships I had made in

LA. Both were gorgeous, savvy city girls who followed career paths. Both were perfectly preened and together weighed as much as I currently did. Both were also child-free.

It was another sparkling Sydney day and I wanted to be by the harbour to take a moment and breathe in its beauty. I could only imagine what life would be like weeks from now lugging a baby around.

I had only just seen Renae the previous May when I was in LA collecting my belongings from the storage unit. My trip there was just a quick one but we managed to squeeze in a last minute drink at a bar in Venice Beach, my old stomping ground. I hadn't really divulged too much about my Make-A-Baby mission so it was crazy that just eight months later, I was sitting opposite her in Sydney with a fully grown bubba in my belly. As a citizen of the globe, she just so happened to fly into Sydney days earlier to escape Cali's cold. It seemed serendipitous that we were both in town at the same time and worthy of a harbourside cheerio.

I hadn't seen my bestie Chelsea in almost two years, which meant she missed the full brunt of the 'Seven Sides of Hayley'. Kind of like Disney's seven dwarfs, only mine related to who was along for the rollercoaster ride of which no-one was at any wheel or operating any switch. There was Phoenix The Phantom, Ms. Erable, Ataloss, Seed McQueen and Shan Choosy to name a few.

She embraced me with an armful of baby gifts, which felt odd to have my hands on this type of merch in a bar. How times had changed! It was December 31, 1999 when I partied the second millennium away in this exact location taking in the most magnificent snap, crackle and pops of colour above the bridge and across the harbour. I contentedly smiled as I reminisced party days of past. Oh, how I definitely felt ready to do this city in a whole new motherly way. Hug her tight with a whole lot of bosom.

We nattered away for about an hour over drinks, talking and giggling about our former lives in LA. Renae had just been dating some guy in the UK, but decided he was too annoying to continue a relationship with. There was always some dude on the scene, but none were ever FB pic or 'status update' worthy. Those days now seemed like a lifetime ago.

As the afternoon's glow faded, the girls decided they'd prefer to shift locations and slide into a spot with a little more social atmos. We followed the walkway under the harbour bridge across to Kirribilli that had me push an extra seventeen kilos of belly up a hill. It was quite the change from the last time I was here with Chels and my faux pregnancy.

We decided on an outside table at one of Kirribilli's busy eateries and ordered pizza, and water before we had even parked our posteriors. The moment our food arrived, the three of us hoovered down our first slices. Then, out of the late afternoon blue, a gloomy cloud emerged along with the winds of change.

I had just taken a bite of my second pizza slice, when all of a sudden, questions about my pregnancy were hurled at me like arrows at a close range target. The weathercock just swung from North to South.

*"Hayley, how the hell are you actually going to support this child on your own?"*

*"What if 'baby dadda' comes for his child?"*

*"What if you sell your book and become really wealthy and then 'baby dadda' comes for you?"*

*"Have you got a legal contract in place?"*

*"What about his genetic history?"*

*"Do you know the risks of having a baby at your age?"*

At eight months pregnant, almost ready to pop, it seemed a little late for these questions to be fired at me. My immediate reaction was to take a defensive position. Confused as to why they seemed to be unsupportive of my decision.

As I chewed on what was a light crisp margarita pizza, it didn't mean I couldn't taste the unsavouriness of JUDGEMENT now peppered all over it. These women had chosen, or at least accepted, the child free option. So, why did it matter that I pursued this path? I wondered if they were in fact referring to themselves and their own choices, not so much mine.

It was only now that I connected the dots with what Chelsea had blurted out earlier between drinks. She had said that she had a lot of resentment towards her parents for deciding to have children when they couldn't afford them. My natural reaction was to slap down her declaration but I knew that wouldn't have had an impact. She was comparing me to her situation. Fifty years on, she was still burdened by her upbringing, which had nothing to do with me, then or now.

With great restraint, holding back a strike with a Scorpio sting, I maturely opted to take on a more considerate position. Realising they could not understand my journey as they had not participated in any part of the plot. Sure, I was taken aback at first, but they have a right to their opinions and concerns. It hurt being in the firing line, but I knew they weren't alone with their thoughts and I would be foolish in believing so.

I realised, in that instant, though, that two of my sacred Sista's had defected on me. Or to be fair, I had on them. Regardless of who was the culprit, there was no going back. Our friendships were in the midst of change. Gone would be the days of debaucherous oblations and impromptu evening escapades. Even while I still only had a bun in the oven, I was no longer a childless chick. I was no longer one of them. I had taken it upon myself to change the way we connected.

*"Friends show their love in times of trouble, not in happiness."*
*- Euripides, Greek Playwright and Poet*

Their biggest concern for so many people is collectively: cha-ching—money. So I hit that one straight up:

The idea that people need to be financially secure to procreate is an interesting one, considering so many of us aren't, or will ever truly be, in a position to have children. What does financially secure look like anyway? Does it mean financially free or just able to manage the cost of living? Do either of these two lifestyles look the same to you as they do to me? Some people absolutely can't imagine a life without monthly mani's and pedi's or daily cappuccinos and bagels from their local cafe.

Some people must drive a certain level of car for prestige, to represent a faux economic status. Or live in a certain area and wear certain brands of clothing. Some people wouldn't be able to give any of this stuff up and would be flummoxed at ever entertaining the idea of doing so. They'd rather borrow more cash, work another few hours, and so on, opposed to being "inconvenienced" by not having these unnecessary conveniences or what might be seen by others as "selfish splurges".

Just two years ago the average wage in Australia was about $78,000; it was $31,099 in the USA and £27,000 in the UK. A recent Australian Bureau of Statistics Report showed nearly 30 per cent of Australian households were over-burdened with debt, with mortgages the driving cause. The amount of money people are spending on housing has gone up relative to increases in wages or wage growth.

Soaring costs of living and stagnant wages is a reality across the board. Having a child seems out of reach, on paper, for a good chunk of the population. A pipe dream. So what's the answer? Do we just accept that the affluent have the country's collective permission to breed?

People struggle everywhere. All. The. Time. It's not specific to single mothers. Cities eventually drive a good bunch of us out. The costs to stay amongst the sheeple far outweigh the real cost imposed on our health and lifestyles. I don't believe a single woman abandoning her dreams of raising a family is the resolution. If it means moving to a slower paced, beachy or tree-lined locale on the outskirts of the city to have that absolutely desired child, then so be it. My friend Carmen not only hung up her city skates, she embraced a whole new country way of life. And now she even has the gorgeous child to enjoy it with.

And some might think women who can't afford children shouldn't have them. There are plenty of couples who can't afford them but because there are two of them, does that make it okay? Does that not double the problem? They can be living a credit lifestyle, appearing to own a bunch of materialistic stuff therefore creating a false public status, and because of that, they have more rights than a single woman? Well, that's a warped perception.

I don't go to clubs and bars, dine out often (prefer my cooking anyway), don't enjoy fashion shopping (never have), gamble (other than buy the odd lotto ticket) or even spend my free time dating. Although, perhaps that might be the best way to survive. I have known a few women friends, or should I say acquaintances, who survived by dining out on a man's dime five nights a week—all different dinner dates in rotation week after week.

Finances. It's at the crux of many midlife meltdowns. Throw in the constant pressure of a biological clock, singledom, work wear n' tear, and well, yeah, you have one gigantic hot pot of distress bubbling away.

Carmen knows she "made the choice and the decision to go it alone, but many others haven't been put in that situation where they have HAD to make that decision." She says "I didn't choose to become a single mother. I chose to have a family. I just happened to be single."

I don't think it's that unreasonable to pay $10-15k in a round of IVF using donor sperm as it's handled by many hands before it's finally inseminated. Beyond one cycle however, it becomes very costly, very fast even with a Medicare rebate. Now you have a pain point as you'll likely be throwing away tens of thousands of dollars for a bunch of emotional hell and in many cases, no return.

Carmen's investment with fertility clinics could rival that of a relationship. It had all the traits of one. Emotional ties. Dates. Road trips. Hotel stayovers. Baby making troubles and triumphs. She says "I have NEVER looked at her (my daughter) and thought about the cost. I would do it all again just for her. Well, I did, another eleven times... without success."

"I just see other people who have children, and for many, who are able to become pregnant so easily and readily, and they haven't had to go through all of this and fork out thousands and thousands of dollars to have that child or those children."

It's interesting how mindset surrounding finances aborts children before they can even be made. So despite being an insanely wonderful person, good spirited, kind-hearted, responsible and loving, you shouldn't become a parent because you perhaps aren't as financially stable as you should be? According to who? When did finances take this top position?

Back in the day, wasn't it just about having the security of an income? Sure, many of us can't trust employment these days, but if we really, really wanted to, we can all make money. We don't have to be taken care of by a man who will then allow us to have a child. We shouldn't be chasing men just to use them to secure our paths ahead. No, we should take responsibility for ourselves. If we're not doing that then perhaps this solo motherhood thing is something that should be kept on the 'out of reach' shelf.

Although I do believe we need people breeding to contribute to our economies in the years to come when we need it most, bringing a child into the world and raising them solely on Government assistance is far from ideal. However, there are many people who are not only inspirational but are the epitome of success and apparently defied societal odds. They grew up in poor families or were raised by single mothers.

Their families were dead broke. Extremely poor, yet they ended up okay. No, not just okay. Way more than O fucking K. They've changed-the- world kind of okay. They're incredibly wealthy themselves just in case that point needed any justification. Single motherhood, and even single fatherhood, is no guaranteed predictor of future financial failure for the child, that is for sure.

Oprah Winfrey is a philanthropist, a media mogul and one of the most inspirational souls that ever danced on this planet. Her mother, a teenage girl and single mother, raised her in rural Mississippi. She not only overcame her upbringing hardships, she overcame the trauma of being raped when she was just nine years old.

J K Rowling overcame poverty, single parenthood, a failed marriage, and the loss of her mother to become one of the most influential storytellers of our time. As creator of the iconic "Harry Potter" series, which this woman dreamed up in cafes all around Edinburgh, she is an icon who impacted and touched millions of us around the world with her imagination.

President Barack Obama was born just six months into his mother and father's relationship. His father left the family home to study at Harvard when Barack was still a baby. By the time Barack was two years old, his parents had split up. He spent a handful of years in Indonesia after his mother married her Indonesian partner but came back to Hawaii when he was ten years old. He served two terms as the 44th president of the United States.

Not only a child of immigrants and divorce, the following example was a child with absolutely nothing—not even a home! John Paul Dejoria is a former child of the streets and foster care, gang member and now is a billionaire entrepreneur and philanthropist. He founded the high-end tequila company Patrón Spirits Co. and hair care company Paul Mitchell Systems. The man has a net worth of about $US3.3 billion (in 2018).

Closer to home, Kim was left with a year-old baby in her arms after her husband left her for another woman. Totally in love, she couldn't have fathomed that he would leave her stranded in a city away from her friends and family, totally reliant on his pay cheque while she brought up their baby.

Her friend gave her some money to get on a plane, travel back to her home state and had her move in with her while she got on her feet.

Her ex rarely paid child support so Kim bounced into action and got a job to look after her baby in her new role of single mum. She didn't choose her situation or to be shaken out of marital bliss. It was forced upon her and she made it work. Her daughter has never gone without anything and Kim has never relied on a man to do her work for her.

So finances are not a reason to not be a mother. If I won millions in the lotto tomorrow, does that then give me permission and make me instantly worthy? Would that perhaps give me a rite of passage to still remain or become a shitty, irresponsible, lazy person with chronic addictions loaded with cash. Then will it be absolutely OK to have a child?

A lot more goes into parenting than ca-ching $$$. Besides, no-one knows what's around the corner. Both men and women can be over extended on mortgages or leased up to the wazoo on cars, furniture, home remodels, etc. They're stressed out, unhappy and living a lie. I dunno about you, but I wonder what kids learn in those types of environments. I ain't gonna fudge it....sure, money most definitely helps.

Love and cuddles are priceless. They are basic child necessities that don't require a credit card. If you got them to give, can put food on a table and a roof over your head for eighteen years, then it's very likely YOU CAN DO THIS. You'll figure it out and be OK. So too will the kiddies.

Many men feel the same financial pains that women do. I've been told that's why many delay having babies until a lot later in life. They're essentially providers, a role bestowed on them whether they like it or not and want or need to be set up in order to do just that—provide. They also know that their career goals and financial plans don't necessarily coincide with a woman's biological timeframe. I'm fairly certain this is why some men don't take the baby leap and women find themselves duped in their relationships; because although they want children, they're not able to make the commitment without all their ducks in a row.

I'm a smart, strong, responsible, ambitious, perceptive, emotionally aware and caring woman. I'm not some fool that just thought this idea up without deep consideration. My mum raised two children on her own.

I chose to be who I am today and have travelled the path I have because I found inner strength and courage to forge ahead despite my hardships and screw ups. Would I have loved a helping hand here and there? Sure. A mentor and role model to show me the way? Hell yes. But I am here now without having had that.

I had placed expectations on my last relationship to finance a chunk of my life. It was a life of constant financial stress. As soon as I stopped living a life according to someone else, I instantly became richer in my own life. So while my bank account doesn't have the digits I would love to see, I am so wealthy in life, love, friendships and freedom. Fact: I know I'll always be OK and my child will not miss out on a thing. That is me stepping up and not expecting to be saved. It's me being a woman in modern society. This is the kind of attitude that comes at no cost.

Laura was one such financially focused woman I spoke with who is caught up with moving forward based on the same two things that held me up. Love and money. She told me she felt such self-doubt and road blocked because of finances. As a Canadian living in Australia, where she now calls home, she's worried about being alone a country without a solid support system.

"I could go back home to do this (have a baby solo), but I am happy in Australia. I'm almost forced to choose it. To me it's more of the constant internal questioning, "Can I make it work here? Do I have to go home?" Then at that point, I go into a spiral where I say holy fuck is my life really at this point? Is this seriously happening?!"

She continues, "it's that feeling of a tornado effect where I am practical; where I can do this, this, this and this and it's going to happen but then you realise the sad part of it, which is I have to do this. It's almost like you're mentally gearing yourself up to take that next step.

Like anything, whether it is a job, how much you're going to spend on a vacation. You're gearing yourself up to committing to something pretty big and it's probably one of the biggest commitments you could do."

Yes, a 'kid kitty' is a great idea but they're not always easy to commit to. So too is having an emergency bank account - but how many of us have those and constantly topped up? The reality——most of the population is in debt. It's how society functions. And here's the filthy well-kept secret. We're the rule, not the exception.

*"But how are you going to support your child?"*

This was the real underlying question. This decision was given A LOT of thought. It wasn't an accidental pregnancy or as a first preference to do it alone. As an educated, entrepreneurial, now 42-year-old professional with a 'do whatever it takes' attitude, I did not have a baby to settle for a life on welfare.

Aussies are blessed to have access to the Family Support Program, which is there to ensure the wellbeing and safety of children. Its tax-free benefit extends to a large chunk of the nation's family households who earn what can be considered a middle-class income.

Its purpose is to be a supplement for some, a bridge gap for others, or an olive branch for either singles or couples so they can spend some invaluable time with their precious young child/children. It is not intended to be a way for people to avoid working and not contribute to society. Those taxpayers' dollars are for assisting in the raising of children, not for living a full-time bludger lifestyle. Denmark or Norway would be a much better residential option for taking advantage of that!

Using a private donor opposed to a clinic has meant that the money I would have spent in a fertility clinic, has now been re-assigned to raising my child. I'm also blessed to have the hands of many in my village. Their second biggest concern seemed to be my age, more specifically, the problems, issues and the potentially dire consequences of having a baby over forty.

I did consider the 'what if there is a birth complication' thought. What if something went wrong? If the baby was born with a defect, how could I afford a child that would perhaps need constant medical care? I lamented over this. I chose to focus on the flipside and hope for the best possible outcome—a healthy child. The rest wasn't in my hands and I would do everything and anything I could to help a child in need. If I found a way to have a baby, then I sure as hell would find a way to ensure that baby would get the care required.

I know I can give a child the right kind of environment to thrive. There are a thousand ways to achieve the same result. Sure, it takes a whole lot of effort to put a child in the best position possible to succeed in life; it also takes a strong-willed woman to grab a machete and shred out her own path.

Some other concerns I was bombarded with that night included:

*"Baby Dadda is gonna come to get your bubba!"*

No, he's not and here's why. Mr Stork has his own child. He also has 3 other donor children. He does not want mine. He does not want to fight me to change stinky nappies, spend hours on end hanging about in playgrounds, add more day-care and school drop-offs and pick-ups to his day, juggle his own family life with another three women and their lives, give me or the other mothers a huge chunk of his weekly wage, pay for school uniforms, have my child and his friends over for sleepovers x 3, help with homework or baby sit.

No, he wants his own life. He doesn't want to relocate his life to Queensland and disrupt his family and work life. Nor does he want to give us access to any family inheritances or drain his superannuation.

Does he want to know how my child is and for my child to know who he is? Absolutely! And so he should. My child shares his DNA. They will forever be genetically tied. We are "friends". He gifted me a child and I want him to be known in my boy's story when my child is ready to invite that. If my child wants his DNA dadda to come over for dinner, then he will have a place setting at the table.

I don't buy into the fear that all men would help someone have a child and then want to ruin everyone's lives by fighting for rights of that child. I'm sure it happens, but I bet many of those are because that man has either played a daddy role and then had the situation changed on him or the couple were romantically involved. When there is an emotional connection, then there is more room for error. A straight up amicable, adult exchange is less likely to incite that.

If ever his intention changed at some point in my child's life and he wished for more contact, would it really bother me too much? If he wants to make that effort, then that's fine. At the end of the day, my LO (little one) will be calling those shots.

Besides, would my baby dadda dare take on a bunch of women? No smart or stupid man would dare.

*"What about the legalities? Have you considered those?"*

What's illegal about hooking up with someone? Or even having a roll around in a haystack? Nothing! What about accepting some cash for doing so?

Well, as it's been mentioned it's prohibited around the world to pay or receive payment for sperm. Restrictions are in place mainly to prevent inbreeding or accidental consanguinity between donor siblings. If you do pay to receive sperm through NI you'd most likely be under a different set of laws of which sexual services are defined by and another one for buying a 'cup o sperm'.

Stephen Page, who is an internationally recognised family lawyer based in Australia, recommends donors and recipients follow a process prior to picking up a fresh jar.

He insists these three things should happen:

- There should be extensive, meaningful discussions between parties about their respective roles. There shouldn't be three or more shades of grey.
- They should have comprehensive counselling with a fertility counsellor, typically a psychologist who is a member of the Australia New Zealand Infertility Counsellors Association (ANZICA). There are some fertility counsellors in private practice and others associated with IVF clinics.
- There should be a sperm or other donor agreement in place.

*"Did you sign a legal contract?"*

We discussed so many things and by doing so we were able to establish, very early on, if he was an ideal donor for me and if I was an ideal recipient for him. I had him sign a preconception agreement that we fleshed out together signed with his pseudonym. I didn't use a lawyer or have an official legal contract drafted. As a single woman, the government expects me to exhaust all avenues in finding "the father" so they can chase him for mandatory child support payments. As a donor, he gifted me with sperm to create my child. He did that for me, not with me. He did not have any intention and still does not have any desire to be a parent of my child.

Our letter of intention outlined both our expectations of how the donorship would evolve once the baby arrived. It highlighted that we both acknowledged and agreed that the donor "provided his semen for the purposes of said artificial insemination and did so with the clear understanding that he would not demand, request, or compel any guardianship, custody or visitation rights with any child born from the home insemination procedure."

We both agreed that I would not hold the donor legally, emotionally or financially responsible in any way for the child. If I decided to add another child to my family, that would be discussed at a later date, but in no way was that possibility an obligation for the donor. I made it clear to him that all things related to my child were my responsibility. Such as name, religion, schooling, or who a guardian may parent my baby alongside me or perhaps take full custody if something tragic ever happened to me.

Mr Stork acknowledged and understood that he would not have any paternal rights whatsoever with my child. Even though a preconception agreement or donor contract may not be a legally binding document, I believe they're crucial for moving forward along the donor route. Mr Stork, aka the biological father and I needed to clearly outline the boundaries and expectations for both of us with my child's life at the core of those decisions.

We agreed that if we ever disputed any of these terms that we would discuss our alternate views as opposed to handing over cash to lawyers. Not that I believe we will ever go down that path, but I am also astute and aware that we are human and humans do change their minds. So remaining open and flexible is how I have approached this. Managing both our expectations was, and is crucial. We were in such agreement from the get-go I haven't felt threatened or in fear in any way throughout this whole process.

As a single woman, this document will not likely hold up in a family court, but it does prove what the conception decision was based on. Hopefully one day, in the not too distant future, the law will recognise the donor as such and therefore protect the solo mother as the only parent. I'm working on it!

I left the father's name blank on the birth certificate as he is never going to parent my child. Same-sex couples and heterosexual couples can add their partner's names down as a parent. As a single woman, without a partner, I will be taking care of my child 100 per cent. Single women who use donors are in a minority group and the law still doesn't have our backs just yet. If I was ever to be followed up on, I would be in alignment with the law. Yes, remember, this is the rogue route, and there are a few nuances that need to be carefully manoeuvred to stay on the right side of the law. The way I see it, it comes down to trust. I trusted my donor and built up so much rapport with him that I just knew we had each other's backs.

A side note directed to my sceptic friends—yes, he's a good guy. They do exist as I have proven. Despite me making a point about the various donor types out there, most just want to help women and do not want, nor expect, anything in return other than your happiness. Oh and pictures!

He did request pics of my baby on his birthday, updates on school, a visit here or there if we're in the neighbourhood, and for the child to know who he is and why he exists in our lives at all. As we're maintaining contact, we didn't just exchange Facebook names—I have all his personal details. Facebook owns your page so they have the right to change or delete it if they choose. You need much more than this info from your donor in case these profiles are ever deleted.

I do suggest if anyone wants a full sibling for their child, they use a clinic to freeze some extra sperm as there are no guarantees that you will be able to access more from your donor at a later date. Navigating the nitty gritty legal details may be the hairiest part of this whole path; that's why choosing the right donor is critical. I figured that no matter what type of SHIP anyone enters into, whether it is marriage, de facto partnership or even a business partnership, there is always risk associated with it. Yep, I'm a risk taker so I was prepared to take the risk.

*"What about his genetics?"*

Well, I don't think I have ever asked someone I am madly in love with about their genetics. Then again, other than perhaps, Ian, I was never ready to procreate with anyone. Other than maybe asking a few questions about their families, there is no way I would have asked my Big Loves One and Two about their genetic history. I was far too besotted with both of them. Despite not being ready either time for itty bitty people, any piece of their DNA would have more than delighted me.

Would I have my man genetically tested before saying I do? No. Not if there didn't seem to be anything to be concerned about in his bloodlines. Would I abandon him because he might have some future medical issue? No. I'd marry him anyway. It's no different to my childhood friend Katie who had a mutation in BRCA1, which is one of the breast cancer genes. Being a carrier in no way would have impeded her now-husband Ethan from marrying her. Which obviously it didn't. They've been together for fifteen years and she's only recently undergone a double mastectomy.

Here's a little info on the most common genetic disorders:

Cystic Fibrosis (CF) is a life-threatening condition that mostly affects the lungs and digestive system due to a malfunction in genes related to the exocrine system. This system "glitch" over produces thick and sticky mucus which not only causes the system to struggle to function, but it also traps bacteria creating a haven for it to thrive. On average one in 25 people carry the CF gene—most of whom are unaware that they are carriers. While there is no cure, treatment such as vitamins, exercise and physio can help manage symptoms and improve quality of life for life.

Down syndrome is a common chromosomal abnormality that affects approximately 1 in 1000 newborns (particularly in older expectant mothers), and results when an extra copy of genes occurs on chromosome 21. DS or DNS is caused when there are 47 chromosomes in each cell instead of 46. Although DS can be detected by prenatal testing, babies affected typically show the following features at birth such as decreased muscle tone in the face, developmental delays, and heart and digestive system defects.

Huntington's disease (HD) causes degeneration of the nerve cells in the brain and central nervous system. It's a complex and severely debilitating disease, of which there is no cure, that results in a gradual loss of cognitive (thinking), physical and emotional function.

Sickle Cell Anaemia occurs when red blood cells are unable to carry adequate oxygen throughout the body due to their shape deformation. Healthy red blood cells are shaped like discs, allowing them the flexibility to travel through tight blood vessels. However, with SCA, the red blood cells have an abnormal crescent shape resembling a sickle. This means they don't easily move through some blood vessels causing a blood blockage and restricting flow throughout the body. This extremely painful disease is most common in people of African and Mediterranean Backgrounds.

Thalassemia is another blood disorder common to people of African and Mediterranean descent. It affects haemoglobin production, which in turn causes severe anaemia. Haemoglobin is found in red blood cells and carries oxygen to all parts of the body. Organs become starved for oxygen and are unable to function properly when haemoglobin supply is affected.

Tay-Sachs disease mainly affects people of French Canadian and Eastern European Jewish descent. It's a disorder that is caused by a faulty gene which is supposed to produce an enzyme crucial to the health of the brain and spinal cord. Without it, the nerve cells in the brain and spinal cord destruct causing paralysis. Life expectancy of a child with Tay-Sachs is usually less than five years.

Fragile X Syndrome affects men more so than women, causing developmental problems including learning disabilities, behavioural challenges and mild to moderate intellectual disability as well as certain physical characteristics. This condition is caused by a change in the FMR-1 gene which helps create a protein required for healthy brain development.

It is also the most common single-gene cause of autism worldwide. A recent case in Australia had a family sue Genea, the country's premier provider for fertility, IVF and other assisted conception treatments, as the couple's two children were born with Fragile X despite the mother having had a test to confirm that she was not a carrier. Unfortunately, the test was wrong, as she did, in fact, have Fragile X. They reached a settlement in November 2017 for a lump sum.

Haemophilia is when the blood doesn't clot properly causing a person to suffer from continual blood loss through an injury. This can be highly dangerous and means that what may be a scrape of an elbow, which is considered a minor accident for anyone else, can become life-threatening for those with the disease.

Muscular dystrophy (MD) encapsulates a range of rare diseases all caused by genetic abnormalities. Each one of them attacks body muscles in varying degrees causing their functionality to progressively decline. The level of pain and symptoms may start straight out the gate in babies or develop slowly over time. Some people are born with a mild form of MD which develops over time and doesn't lead to serious disability. With management, a healthy lifestyle and positive outlook on life, mild MD can come along for a very long and fulfilling life ride but just not rule it. To be at risk of passing a trait onto your child, both you and your partner need to be carriers of the same recessive genetic disorder. If this occurs, there is a one in four chance that your child will be born with that disorder.

The reality is, it's not uncommon that you are blissfully unaware you are a carrier of a recessive genetic disorder. This is because it has no identifiable impact on your own health. However, on average, many people will be a carrier of at least one genetic variation.

Once I had more awareness about the more common genetic disorders, having been educated through the clinic and in doing my own research, it became much more important in how I selected sperm for my child. The donor route had me prioritising and making decisions based on medical history and genetics above physical features. As I wasn't emotionally attached to who would be the biological father of my child, I paid more attention to the things I otherwise wouldn't have.

My donor list wasn't about ticking off a list of qualities that I'd like in a relationship because I wasn't looking for a partner. I was looking for the right characteristics and genetic material to create a child. I wanted strong genes to maybe even counteract my more ordinary and less flattering DNA traits. Fortunately, Mr Stork had done some genetic testing and was not a carrier for common diseases and/or disorders. I wasn't a carrier either.

Other wish list items included: Strong physical features. A sensitive soul. An honest person. Someone free from mental illness (in case my DNA has something), who was donating for the right reasons, had his own family life and someone who would be part of my extended family with other siblings with other families. I didn't want to birth lots of babies so knowing there were a few other siblings (but not a football team) out there who were healthy and normal, was a bonus for me. I also needed my donor to be accessible and known to my child from birth.

*"What if you sell your book and baby dadda wants a piece of the action?"*

This book wouldn't exist without baby dadda. Word. In fact, this book wouldn't exist without ANY of the people who participated in my pregnancy journey.

*"Why be a single mother by choice?"*

I, like my friend Carmen, chose to be a mum; I didn't choose to be single, but however that looks in due course is still to be revealed. I also think I'm a solo mother by circumstance, not so much one of choice. For me, I don't see why it's so farfetched for so many women to decide on becoming mothers without the biological father by their sides. It cuts out so much emotional BS and women are more than able. So the stigmatisation of single mothers needs to stop. Times have changed, people! Single women are also not all destined to be single for the rest of our lives - if we so choose!

*"What if you regret it if you proceed solo?"*

What if I regret it if I don't? There was a moment on one particular day when I visualised rolling out my life. It was mapped out on architectural sized drawing paper that I threw across a large table to view. I looked my timeline over and lamented what it looked like both with and without me being a mother. I felt such different physical reactions to both. One being 'cup half full'; the other, the child-free version, was half empty.

While I was working in Tasmania and while filming a story at an upmarket hostel, I met a lovely woman not too much older than me who was also there on business. The following morning, after chatting for a few hours over dinner at the communal table, she asked how old I was.

"Forty," I proudly responded.

She was like, "Oh, you're at that tricky age." She could totally smell the distinct scent of deeper despair; it was familiar to her.

I told her I was very recently back to being a sleeping starfish in the middle of the bed. She enquired about kids. I said it was a concept that was swirling about in the abyss of going nowhere land. She told me she and her husband pondered it when she had hit the same crisis point. She wanted kids. Him not so much.

He did concede a little by having his sperm tested to see if it could at least sow seed. That was the most life a baby between them lived. It lived and died as a baby idea. She then got a great job and threw herself into work. Their life went on and he never brought it up. Now she was in the midst of separating from him.

I asked her if she wished she made it happen or prioritised differently. She responded, "I'm 51. I wonder what my life would be like with a nine or ten year-old. I should have done it. Now my marriage is gone and my chance for that has, too." It was some more divine timing to sprinkle over my almost over cooked eggs simmering away in my pressure cooker.

My Mum recently told me a story about one of her close friends and her husband choosing not to have children. They retired early and relocated to a stunning property in Pemberton, Western Australia, which had multiple guest rooms spread amongst a huge cottage garden.

They were ready to live their fabulous life—entertain, travel the planet, enjoy sleep-ins and tend to their acres of gardens. After only two weeks of moving in, she found her husband dead on the garage floor. He had died from a heart attack. They were just starting to enjoy a life on their terms; a life they had saved for but the one they had planned for was cut short. She has now sold her dream property and had to rewrite how her Life's Third Act plays out solo.

I didn't have my child just to have someone, a stop gap when I grew old. These stories did resonate however. It seemed most women I knew who didn't have children, not the ones who were affected due to medical reasons, did indeed want to be mothers. It's not like they consciously chose not to have them. Rather, 'not having them' just kind of happened.

Tracey concurs. I met her through a friend when I was on a video shoot not long before I wrapped on writing this book. I was enthralled by her story to fall pregnant and have babies ten years later than me. It blew my mind how she changed her solo course in the nick of time.

At 51, she had missed the boat to have kids but somehow miraculously managed to cast out a life line and land a life raft. She told me that she didn't deliberately seek out being a career woman, or chose work over having kids. She was just "doing it". Then when her relationship hit the skids and the future of family looked bleak, she found herself working her way through the typical single woman thought phases. "First it was 'I will never have kids unless it's with my true love, if I can't have a child naturally I'll accept it as it wasn't meant to be, I would never choose to do this on my own, I would never do IVF—it's not for me'. Then eventually you find yourself here."

She blames the sexual revolution of the 60s for the mess we're in. "It failed so many of us and not just women." Prior to this social movement it was the done thing for a young man to ask a young woman out. They courted. They married and had kids. She thinks this 'try before you buy' approach has let us all down big time.

Just in my case alone, she has a well-founded point. Marriages declined and divorce rates skyrocketed. So too did those pesky STI's. The traditional family foundation got a shake up while young peeps got their free lovin' shake on.

Feminism and the introduction of birth control pills and latex condoms inspired these new behaviours and attitudes towards casual sex. Having multiple partners became socially acceptable outside the strict confines of heterosexual marriages. The childbearing years could be pushed to some other time and jumping straight into marriage with the high school sweetheart was somewhat given a social slap by peers.

These days while we're busy figuring out life and love simultaneously, we're being distracted from noticing time and how it's gobbling up our chance to become mothers. "Oh they'll (kids) come...but they don't just come" she said. Fortuitously though, they did for her. "I went to speak to my doctor and asked for a fertility test thinking she just filled out the paperwork to amuse herself. To my surprise she didn't balk at my request. Had she not given me the go ahead to do a test I probably wouldn't have pursued it further." Tracey completed two cycles of IVF using donor eggs and at 52 became the mother of twin girls. She was quick to reiterate that her story is most definitely an exception and not the rule; that waiting is a risky game to play.

As I listened to her, it had me ponder the idea that perhaps both nature and nurture had nothing to do with my single woman predicament. The sexual revolution is the cunning perpetrator. Grabbing the destiny wheel to become a single parent is at first intimidating. For me, the decision evolved into empowerment. Sure, there's no hunky husband or hot partner on the scene (yet) but there's also no in-laws, and for some of us, that would be sublime.

"*What about marriage?*"

Marriage or what I refer to as 'mirage' is something I find so elusive, foreign and as far as I can see, most definitely doesn't stack up to being what it's marketed as, probably because it's founded on a relationship and as you well know I suck at those.

I'm in good company, too, thank goodness. It seems many of my closest friends struggle when it comes to sticking with their own legally bound partners in crime. Their number ones. Their peps in their steps. Their sunsets on their horizons. Their Shnookums'. Hun Buns. You get the picture. Of my closest ten friends, eight of them are currently wearing their new sexy title of divorcee—one I would happily swap out for 'socially infertile'. Any day!

The D club seems to have a constant queue of peeps lining up to cut ties from the moment the business day starts. It reminds me of the long lines and wasted hours I spent at the DMV on any day and at any hour. Those lines were always filled with vibrant folks and never seemed to dwindle down.

Just in Australia, of the one hundred and fifteen thousand odd couples who leaped into the mirage in 2015, another 43 per cent chose to officially pull the kill switch. A big chunk of those households, about a third if I were to throw out a number, directly impact the little ones in the house.

Up until I was about thirty, there were only a few people I knew who were divorced and they were a lot older than me. Ten years later either that number had increased tenfold or maybe I just removed my blindfold to this reality.

As a teenager, and having been a child of divorce, I didn't see single parenting as anything but normal. Perhaps that's because I never lived between two homes or got caught up in a shared custody showdown.

Many of my friends' parents were together. Sure they may have been in miserable marriages perpetuating the faux 'Leave It to Beaver' happy family image, but they still managed, or at the very least were able to live in the same house together. Again, I saw this as normal. Something that we, meaning us kids, naturally evolved into having or being part of ourselves when we grew up.

*"The separation of a childless couple is dramatic,*
*but the separation of a couple with children is always tragic."*
*- Louis Garrel*

Now, divorcees were not only my age, they were my friends. And their kids were the ones who were often caught up in the crossfire. Three of my closest girlfriends have had to deal with some seriously ugly shit. Some of that ugliness still lingers on some twelve months after they inked their signatures to revoke their original love and honour pledges.

Lorrie and her now ex, Josh, have endured a long custody battle over their two young daughters. She's had the police out a few times to her house when he's arrived unannounced or at her work place causing quite the scene in front of her clients. Belittling and abusing her, it has me wondering if an AVO (apprehended violence order) really has the strength to draw a line and uphold it between broken lovers. Josh was determined to make her life hell, even sending in his mates to hang at her local haunts to rattle her. It's like he had to piss over every place she walked so the pebbles she stepped on were in fact egg shells—his presence felt every step of the way. I am not sure what this was to achieve but it's sad to witness the bright light of a friend's eyes dim down.

My guy friends have dealt with some sucky situations, too. One is currently fighting for full custody of his two children. His ex-wife has moved in with another man and his kids, who are five and three, are struggling with the daddy switch sitch. Once happy-go-lucky kids who lived each day just being kids, now they aren't smiling the way they were born to do. Their eyes reveal what their tongues can't say. No loving parent wants any child of theirs to suffer, yet here they are in a situation they didn't choose to be in.

Unfortunately, the range of emotions every human needs to go through in order to heal from a marriage breakdown can be a painful, long, drawn-out journey, not only for them but for those who are closest to them. It's different for every individual and cannot be dictated by time.

Many men feel duped in their relationships, married or not. Women mostly head to their girlfriends with bottles of wine to whine aka share

TMI. Well, at least for their immediate tension release. Men, on the other hand, tend to head inwards, hang out on their own with their long lost buddy Jack Daniels or use a woman for the night for some female company or release by dialling a 1-800 number or moving from a bar to her bed.

Or they do what some are doing and join the MGTOW Movement, which stands for 'Men Going Their Own Way'. This group, is one of a few that encourages straight men, who have been kicked to the curb and, according to them, financially swindled by women, to avoid them and relationships entirely.

A friend of mine figured out her partner was being enlightened by this mob while they were settling on their divorce and custody terms. His aggressive gibberish toward her allegedly came directly out of this 'manosphere' men's club. Members here actually actively caution men against having serious romantic relationships with women. They especially preach against walking down an aisle and saying, 'I do'.

With many men getting the raw end of the deal in courts, it didn't surprise me that the MGTOW movement exists. The legal systems are more favourable to women and men have a hard task pushing their cases forward. I get it. The playing field doesn't work for everyone and men can in many cases feel the bite much more than their exes. MGTOW operates across a bunch of levels categorised by pill colours depending on how scarred the man is from his break up and how much interaction he continues to have with people who have vaginas.

While I type, I'm saddened by what this relationship landscape looks like. I mean, I'm essentially part of a WGTOW movement (Women Going Their Own Way) without realising it but doing so without all the hostility (I hope). At least I no longer feel as though I'm moving away from something, rather, moving towards it. And I could never deeply despise the entire population of the opposite sex.

Despite the appalling divorce figures, hetero male marriage-hate clubs and frightening family split stats, the idea of marriage still oddly has acquired a cosy, little spot in my occipital cortex. I managed to shake most of the fantasy out of me after my monumental life smack down.

Once I headed down the solo baby route, finding that perfect human to take my hand, lost its significance somewhat. I didn't want to meet someone, get married, and fall pregnant only to then fall out of love, divorce and then fight over what days he could have access to our child.

Packing weekly overnight bags and having to stay connected to my past in order to co-parent just created anxiety and sucked the joy out of wanting to do this with someone. Having a seat watching my friend's theatre play out, I felt I'd end up on the stage, too. It's not the kind of performance I wanted to participate in, and it certainly wasn't the attention I wanted to attract or share with the world. I know it doesn't all turn out this icky, however posts on single parents FB support groups certainly doesn't offer much hope and with my list of bad relationship choices, it seemingly would be inevitable I'd join them.

Fortunately, a teeny bubble of hope remains and I believe I'm not going to die a spinster (unless I was what Bridget Jones refers to in her third flick as a SPILF - Spinster I'd Like to Fuck), and I don't think I, or love, is entirely a lost cause.

I guess you're wondering what my thoughts are on male energy and influence in my life are, yeah?

Well, I love a masculine scent, so male energy is a must for me in my life. Fortunately, they are everywhere in my world. Men are married to my friends. My girlfriends are dating them. The male species are even my friends. My work colleagues are men. My neighbours next door are young fellas. My regular barista is even a bloke. The guy at the gym is OMG—a guy! My donor, whom I'm friends with, is a man too. I have relationships with men. I plan on dating one again at some point. I'm well aware of what men bring to the table and my little guy will certainly get his daily dose of testosterone.

Now you may wonder if any of my mother friends asked me these Q's?

Yes, a few did, but not in the same tone or manner as a few of my child-free friends did. For the most part, both my close mother-by-choice friends, divorced mother and married mother friends didn't for a moment throw warnings or shade my way. They know what life is like with children and wouldn't wish to deny me that experience. They know I'm a perfectly capable human being who can do this. They also know what I have ahead of me—a baby is full-on 'I know, I know!'. But they also want me to share in the joy that is being a mum.

I think it's healthy to hear the concerns of friends and allow them the space to express objections and worries. But at the end of the day, if they're not supportive or compassionate, perhaps the SHIP has run ashore and it's time to abandon it for a while. And that's OK too.

# Chapter 21
# Man of The House

*"It ain't what they call you, it's what you answer to."*
*- W.C. Fields, actor-comedian*

*I AM NOT SURE WHY* it all of a sudden jumped into my head to change my last name to essentially my pen one, but the more I thought about it, the more it made sense. I didn't want my son to take on the name of my father or the energy that came with it. I wanted fresh new light because that is what I had created, and it was important for me to take ownership of both his and my identities.

Of course, had I exchanged vows with a beloved, I may have taken his name, but I figured since I didn't need to be married to make a child, I sure as hell didn't need to be married to change my name. In fact, I liked it, so I put a ring on it. I'm referring to me. Finally, I backed myself without hesitation. With everything. All of me. I don't need a rock from someone. I already rock.

When I told my friend India, whose name was changed from Michelle, which was one of the most popular names of 1980, that I decided to change my last name she told me there are three main reasons why people change their names:

1 - They are criminals
2 - They are up to something illegal
3 - They're nuts

There was also a fourth reason. Because she could! And that's exactly what I thought. I can. So I did.

If anything, this got more of a response from a couple of friends than me having a baby with a stranger did. One girlfriend thought it was a superficial move, as she felt it didn't dive in deep enough to shake the shit up that needed to. The shift I apparently needed was internal and no new name or 'label' could alter my external energy. What cracked me up after absorbing her hour long rant, she called me back a few days later apologising. She somehow overlooked that she had in fact taken on another identity herself back in high school. Yep, she had conveniently forgotten that she swapped out her real birth name of Sharon to Suzie.

The other friend wrote to me to tell me that she thought the change was weird. I couldn't be arsed responding to let her know I thought it was weird that she had to go out of her way to tell me she thought it was weird.

Second names were primarily created as a way to identify people sometime in the late Middle Ages when township populations grew. People acquired locations or jobs as a second name so they could be distinguished from someone else with the same first name. As far I'm concerned my name probably evolved and changed through people and time so it doesn't really hold a whole lot of sentimental value to me.

Once I cracked this can open a whole bunch of worms spewed out with people telling me that they too had changed their names. Even my Plan C DNA man told me his birth name wasn't actually Pim. Like us name changers, people switch their name for all sorts of reasons.

There are, of course, those couples who marry and want to unite by name, de facto couples who want to commit to one another without signing a marriage certificate, divorcees who either want to reclaim themselves or take claim on a new sense of self.

People may just want to distance themselves or reconnect with family if they've had a falling out. Single mums who find replacement dadda figures may choose to change their children's names to be in alignment with their new family. Mums may feel the need to change both hers and her children's names if she is escaping a former violent relationship, fears for their lives and needs to start fresh somewhere else.

It's not uncommon for individuals to anglicise their name to fit in with social circles, avoid discrimination particularly when looking for work or elevating their careers. Or do the opposite by converting to a selected religion or resuming a former ethnology.

It's no news that performers such as actors and musicians often take up stage names. News Flash; Bruno Mars wasn't birthed by a planet. No, when he landed on terra-firma he was stamped with the name, Peter Gene Hernandez. His personal ID was changed so he wouldn't be stereotyped as a Latin singer.

'Archibald Leach' just doesn't have quite the same leading man pizzazz as the name Cary Grant has. When Archie signed on with Paramount Pictures he took on the new identity of Cary, and once he did, he stepped into being a man of style, who oozed charm and masculine glamour.

Book authors often take on pen names, as do script writers. Individuals and couples are business products themselves these days, so it's not so weird since self-branding has become a thing.

There are soooo many reasons. In 2015, in the USA alone there were 85 thousand reasons why. We don't have to keep the name we were assigned; a name we never chose!

I returned from LA a different person. I'm now a better version of my previous self. I changed my name because it was time for me to take ownership of me. Take responsibility. If I was prepared to go to so much trouble to become a mother, then I needed to shake off any residual

JUDGEMENT and EGO that no longer served me. While still essentially a 'Miss' I now needed to be the mother, not the child. I first moved out of home at seventeen and have pretty much always been on my own blazing my own trail, good and bad. People marry themselves these days and at 42, having gone down this path, I've never felt more like the woman I am supposed to be as I do now. I want to break away from the past. I'm not defined by that story of trauma. Did it touch me? Yes. Did it assist in shaping me? Yes. But it is not me. I am me and my son doesn't need to take any of the past on. He can move forward afresh and carve out his own path and define what it is to be a Hendrix.

So, how did I arrive at the surname Hendrix? Plan C Pim, that's how!

Not only would he have been able to offer some great DNA for a bambino, he is the person that inspired the name change to his. It isn't to honour some rock n roll god at all. Pim is a person who I could only hope my boy could resemble even in the smallest way.

He has a huge heart, is open-minded, a global citizen, creative, spiritual, smart, fun, gregarious and has lived his life for him, on his terms. This man played full out, and still does, in every way. He was always someone you'd put on your party invite list. I take my hat off to him for being a radiator of love, life and laughter. We're connected as friends already. Now, in name too.

We met through the Aussie Posse in Hollywood not too long after I flew in. He'd been living there for about ten years before I showed up. So it was great when my sorry arse landed back in Oz that he arrived with his intact not too long after. We both found ourselves along the beach in Byron Bay scratching our heads in unison as we came to terms with reuniting with our mothership.

While I often joked about his good swimming stock, I never attempted to dive in and harvest those pearls. I guess there was a fear that he would say 'no' or the opposite of the spectrum, fall so in love with his child that our friendship would change and as a result, my parenting arrangement would too. I also didn't want to feel that I couldn't choose where I wanted us to live, or maybe travel to for extended periods of time without considering him and his connection with his DNA child.

Again, with so much ' in my head' chit-chat, I decided I wanted less emotional connection with the child's father. A connection, yes, but not one that would infiltrate my world so heavily or rupture his own head and heart with father guilt.

Just loving this man for who he is and having made the decision that I wanted to break free from my own family history of darkness, I decided that Hendrix was a rad last name for my unborn child. So while I didn't get his sperm, I did take his name. A name I'm also proud to put on my book.

I did a quick name-meaning search on Google which revealed that:

"Hendrix is a surname stemming from Henry. The name Henry comes from the ancient Germanic personal name Heimirich from the elements "heim" meaning "home" and "rīc" meaning "ruler, power"."

I didn't know this meaning when I first decided to use it. Once I uncovered this information, though, it reassured me it was perfect for us.

My little witchetty grub would be our man of the house.

## Willing and Able

There was a wave macabre that came over me at around week 24. While my little bundle was still kickboxing my insides, my motherly instinct was kicking ass too. I was overwhelmed with grim thoughts...wondering what if something tragic happened to me?

What if I was in a car accident and I didn't survive but my growing baby did? Like kangaroo road kill, would emergency services reach into my pouch and save my baby? Babies at around this stage have a high chance of surviving and if I wasn't around to care for my newborn, then who would be?

I made an appointment with the public trustee office closest to me to legally clarify what I wanted my end of life plan to be, most importantly, to lay the foundation for the little person who was thrusted to start theirs earlier than anticipated. As a single woman, and a soon to be swinging solo mother, it was imperative I made it clear how life could look for this precious new life if I wasn't to be around. If ever there was a timely moment to create a Will, then this was it. No longer was my life just about me.

Who, if not me, would be the next best in line choice to take care of my unborn son? My brain shuffled through names and images of friends like I was walking my fingers through an old rolodex. Not only would they need to have the capacity to extend care and affection, but to love my child as their own. They needed to possess a similar outlook on life as me, be able to provide a home that wasn't just a place of refuge but a place where ideas can be cultivated, encouraged and hold space for him. To see and hear him.

I pondered potential guardians just as if I were tasting fancy wines. Oh they're 'sweet, soft, light and airy'. He has 'legs, which are helpful limbs, bold, and smooth.' Together they are 'clean, fresh, fruity and lively acidic'. Hmmm then there's these guys––they're 'established, rich and smooth'. Anyone with 'fruity notes' were crossed off the list. So too, big undertones and dirty finishes. I was looking for that perfect blend. One that was well balanced, vibrant, earthy, with lots of personality and, preferably, chemical free.

My mother would only be able to manage with a wee little one with lots of support. I wanted her to have open access without wearing herself out. I considered where my friends currently were in their lives and if a child would be a burden or fit in well into their lifestyles. I considered their financial situation, children, age, values as well as mental and physical health too.

I sipped an icy cold ginger beer as I consulted with a few friends and further deliberated what the bigger picture would look like without me in it. What would be the right fit for him as well as them? What was important for his future? It was a big decision that required some fizz to massage the mind. And even though my substituted alcoholic beverage wasn't what I was gagging for, it was a hit of light and bubbly to get me through the morbid thoughts. It was a fabulous substitute just as my guardians would be for bubs.

I decided on three different friends with the least emotionally vested one to act as executor. Two couples had already volunteered themselves which thankfully made so much sense. Then once I had confirmed approval from everyone, I added their names to the legal documents.

These selected friends are also interchangeable so if their situations change at a later stage, I can easily replace them with someone who might make a better fit.

## Chapter 22

# In the Present with My Present

*"Babies are such a nice way to start people."*
*- Don Herold, writer and cartoonist*

### The Perfect Hatchling

My mum arrived from Perth a few days before I was due at the hospital. It was the same day I received a call from one of the young midwives asking if I would be interested in using a balloon as a relatively non-invasive way of opening my cervix to encourage labour.

WTF? She told me that they would be able to insert it in at the hospital and then I'd be able to go home until I naturally went into labour, which may take a few days. I straight out responded with a, "Hell, no."

Once I was checked into the hospital I wasn't planning on leaving without my little guppy (which just so happens to also be appropriately (called a million fish).

As a 'geriatric', it was expected I'd be induced. I didn't get caught up in the medical reasoning for having to do so, such as placental insufficiency,

I was ready for my 'medium-well done' juicy grub to make his grand entrance into the world. I wanted it to be as swift as possible.

The monks were left off this birth plan. So, too, were the doula, gospel choir, a breath consultant, energy healer, and hypnobirthing practitioner.

Kumbaya tunes and crystals were not welcome, either. Nor was a bathtub so big that my wing women, mother and midwives could all fit in alongside me while I was sure to be wailing. I'm a free spirit and, obviously open-minded, but in this instance, I wasn't up for birthing like a boss. Here I was labelled a geriatric and according to the online dictionary this meant I was 'decrepit; very old or outdated'. Therefore, I required special care.

I just wanted a healthy baby, however which way he was going to be delivered. Preferably I'd be in a hospital bed attended to by a tall, gorgeous, single, middle aged, straight, male doctor. I was actually happy that my little mister would be out a week early as he'd been driving me batty with his non-stop hiccupping night after night.

It was a Friday afternoon when Mum, Kim and I went to the hospital to get me settled. I was taken up to a communal ward where I was to lounge about until later that evening when a nurse would chauffeur me to a suite to insert some prostaglandin gel. This would help bring on labour. When this first lot of gel didn't work they inserted more the following day. There were no signs of change all day. Just different faces of women coming in with bumps and leaving hours later with their bubs.

I was a little surprised that none of the doctors or midwives questioned my single status. It was perhaps the pink elephant in the room but because I had bed side companions, it seemingly didn't draw inadvertent attention to the apparent gaping hole. Either that, or the staff just thought Kim was my partner or maybe I was the girls' surrogate? Or they could very clearly read between the non-verbalised lines?

Early in the evening on my second night, a woman was checked into the bed opposite me. We both had our curtains drawn so we couldn't see one another. I desperately wanted to make conversation with her but didn't know what the ward etiquette was so stayed out of sight in my own personal compound, peeking through intermittently, hoping we'd randomly connect eyeballs so she'd feel compelled to have a natter. I had no idea what to expect with birth. It was all so surreal that I was about to push a kid out and I wanted to talk it out with someone, anyone. Perhaps she could give some last-minute wisdom to this old, apprehensive 'dear in the headlights'.

Hours later, curled up in my single bed with my blankie pulled up over my face to shield me from the cool air-conditioned wind blasts, frightening cries tore through the quiet hospital halls. Half dazed, I switched into 'holy crap, there's a psycho on the loose' mode with my mind immediately moving to 'I hope all the main entry doors have been locked.' The galling screams continued and were soon teamed with banging on the walls. The sounds had me curled up and squealing like fingernails screeching across a chalkboard. The commotion, now just outside my doorway, got louder. I brazenly got up to be a sticky beak and found nurses frantically moved about. They were all too distracted to look in my direction and throw me a bone for comfort. So I shuffled my big butt and belly back to my teeny bed for one, jumped in and hid under the covers.

I awoke to another round of poking and prodding around 6am. Still traumatised by the sounds of the night before, I asked one of the nurses what the pandemonium was all about. She told me a woman had had her baby on the bathroom floor next door. Clearly I'd watched far too many B grade horror flicks as a teen. It was the obvious answer, but it didn't detract from the spookiness of it all. I mean, the set-up, props, eerie sounds and suspense certainly made for a perfect movie scene.

However, it was one I didn't buy a ticket for. That evening, I was taken to the birth suite where I spoke with a doctor about returning home as this baby didn't seem to want to come out. She didn't like that idea. Neither did I just a few days ago; I had been so unflinching when the midwife suggested I could go home once the balloon had been inserted, but now I was a couple of days in. Women had come and gone with their newborns. Me? I was still there. The doc proposed I try once more with the gel before making my decision. She whacked another lot up my hoo-ha, then guided me and my slime smothered vagina off to bed.

It was six thirty the following morning when I woke up desperately needing to use the loo. As I waddled to the bathroom door, liquid poured down my pyjama pants over my ankles and onto the floor. I slid the final two metres as if I was on a slip-n-slide in a last ditch effort to reach the toilet bowl to empty the remaining contents there.

I then alerted the midwives to let them know my water had broken everywhere but into the toilet bowl then apologised profusely for my sticky mess. They chatted with me for a few moments figuring out an action plan as the contractions were kicking in. They decided it was time to take me to a birthing suite.

"Finally!" I hailed. I requested an epidural then quickly contacted Kim and Chez to let them know that now 36 hours later, we were finally in action. Straight out of the gate, the contractions were strong and they only intensified as the minutes passed. The feeling of having my pelvis separate was horrendous. I dreaded each pulse. The girls flew across town to be by my side. They did their best to comfort me, with Kim hydrating me with water and Chez massaging my legs, but each time a wave of pain came I wanted to run away and cry. As I found out, there's nowhere to hide during labour.

Screams were ricocheting through the walls from a woman next door, which were again hard to grasp. Hearing her cries while dealing with my own gushes of excruciating pain had me commiserating for her. Then somewhere in amongst my state of blur, Dr. Dope, the anaesthetist arrived.

I cried, "Where the hell have you been? tears of joy" having waite two and a half torturous hours for him to show up with that needle of relief. In between inhaling gas, I asked if he could help my neighbour, too. My call for pain relief came in just before hers and he could only get to one of us. With hormones flinging about like numbered balls in an air-mix lotto machine, this news made me feel incredibly guilty. I felt I probably could have endured the pain a little longer in order to get her relief.

Those thoughts however were swiftly interrupted when the next big wave crashed down on me. Sucking on gas didn't seem to do much other than distract me from the intense pain of my body splitting in two. It took about another 30 minutes for his epidural handy work to kick in and give me some relief. Those last few contractions, while waiting for the Syntocinon (oxytocin), weren't easy to get through. My dropped bottom lip could have rivalled any toddlers.

Once calm was restored in the suite, I noticed next door had gone quiet too. Turns out, she went from 5 cm dilation to 10 cm in ten minutes and had her baby au natural. I can't, but can, imagine how that felt. I felt very guilty for leaving her to go through that alone. On the flipside, I'm sure she was thrilled she did it on her own.

I, on the other hand, was now riding the oxytocin wave. The drug was delivered automatically. If I needed extra feels, I could just press for more.

As my witchetty grub hadn't progressed south, he was aptly re-nicknamed 'Wombat'. He'd burrowed so high it would have been easier to dislocate my jaw, flip my head back just like 'Mr Reach' famously did in 'Flip Top Head' toothbrush commercial from the 80's, and birth him out of my mouth. For almost another eleven hours, I stayed hooked up to the drip before the delivery doctor could see me and examine how I was doing.

Mum had just arrived at the hospital when he shared his disappointing findings. "You're only 4cm dilated." I looked at the three women by my side, who seemed just as disappointed as me. It had already been a long day and I really hadn't progressed much.

He told us my pelvis wasn't doing what it needed to, so I could continue doing what I was doing and hope that it would straighten up closer to labour or I could take him up on his offer for a Caesarean now.

The ladies and I deliberated for maybe 60 seconds. Having heard some emergency C-section horror stories and now fifty hours in, I didn't hesitate in opting for the C.

Once I gave the go ahead, the long drawn out hour-by-hour wait was a thing of the past. The midwives jumped into action to prep for theatre. I was wheeled upstairs with Kim beside me in scrubs. Dr. Dope was on hand to give me a spinal block before rolling me over to the operating table. Some 20 people were in the room, which felt like I was late to a party. In some way I guess it was as I was about to be cut open and pulled a part-y.

Kim held my hand as the labour shakes took hold. I was freezing and I'm sure the sterile room was icy cold too. The temperature felt like it was on par with a mortuary, not that I've ever been in one. It had been 24 hours since I'd eaten, I was parched, and my entire lower half was numb.

I was ready to be sliced open and my world forever changed. It then only took a few minutes before the sounds of a bawling baby drowned out the room chatter. It was the first sounds of my newborn baby. Remy was finally here and I was now able to reveal his name.

One of the longest secrets I've ever kept.

# Chapter 23
# Genetic Connections

*"The way you help heal the world is you start with your own family."*
*- Mother Teresa*

*Approximately 75 percent of all surveyed donor offspring would recommend that parents use a known or willing-to-be-known donor*
*– Donor Sibling Registry*

THIS IS PART THREE OF this mission. One was becoming exceedingly fertile and securing semen. Two was staying highly nourished throughout the pregnancy and giving birth to a healthy baby. And now this is the third part...the child's perspective and their right to know how they were conceived and have access to that information.

Part of my donor selection process, and one of the major draw cards for me using a known donor, was the fact that my child would be able to connect with him and his siblings. This is a very important step in this conception route, but it wasn't one I was so in tune with when I started out. My sole mission was to get pregnant—to beat the biological clock and satisfy my only desire: to become a mum. While it was something I thought about, I really didn't focus on its importance until I was pregnant. Then it became my hot topic of conversation with Mr Stork.

He not only has his own child who is a sibling to mine, there are three other women out there with babies, too. It's imperative they know Remy exists as I do not believe in withholding information or telling porky pies (lies). I feel it encroaches upon a child's identity and their rights as humans. It's up to the mothers and ultimately the kids to do what they wish with the information.

For some though, it may just be to let it RIP.

Women who advertise for a donor requesting 'NO CONTACT' may not comprehend the injurious nature of doing so. The fear of their chosen donor infiltrating how they run their lives or will want to participate as a Dad is usually what drives this, however uncommon it is.

Men who donate as private donors generally feel that children need to know who they are so the offspring can avoid identity issues later. They donate to be known donors not unknown ones. It does not mean they want to parent the child but being a part of that child's story is of paramount importance. Just sharing photos, having a social media link and connecting with siblings is often the only type of connection most stipulate.

I personally believe it's detrimental to a child's mental and emotional state to deny them their DNA links. It's actually a conversation that's often instigated by an inquisitive child sooner than a protective parent might possibly consider.

Testimonials from the Donor Sibling Registry reinforce my thoughts on this. They have conducted studies finding that the primary motivation for parents assisting their children in searching for their child's donor siblings was due to curiosity. They found that the reason most donor children wanted to seek out their biological fathers was to enhance their sense of identity. Single mothers were the most likely to support this as well as lesbian couples. Hetero couples were least likely to do so.

The way things are going, it's only a matter of time for the masks worn by all anonymous and secretive known donors are stripped from them and more light is shone over them anyway. Sperm donors who used clinics are being tracked down in multiple ways well before the children turn eighteen (sixteen in some places) thanks to technology and curious kiddies. Accessing unknown donor information was an incredibly arduous process and in most cases finding DNA dads failed. But not anymore. Same applies for locating the kids whether they were conceived using a clinic or not. If other siblings do any of the tests on the market, they can be traced to one another.

Many fertility clinics don't have a thorough birth registry system, so it wasn't until a few independent donor registries, like the Donor Sibling Registry, popped up online allowing parents or their children a way to locate their other donor siblings. By entering the donor ID code into the system, kids can be matched with half-brothers and sisters around the globe. If that doesn't work, they can use the information provided by donors at the clinics to do online Google searches or find them via DNA tests and piecing together family trees.

Caitlin is one such young girl whose mum, Katrina, used donor sperm to conceive her through a clinic. She's always known that her mother used a donor as it was always part of their dialogue. In a conversation with them, Caitlin told me her, "Mum has always told me. And I like that she has always told me cause it lets me know. As long as I can remember, she has always just told me. So I have always just known."

Katrina told Caitlin how she came to be from about the time she was 2 years old. Having heard it so many times, she soon became bored with its repetition. Katrina then opted to incorporate the story through the 'My Story Books' but Caitlin didn't like them. Katrina then got creative and "from then on, made the donor a human being. So every little thing I could glean from the profile was like...Caity likes spicy Thai food. So if we were in a Thai restaurant I'd say it's interesting you like Thai food, because your donor likes Thai food, too."

Turning her donor into a real life person was one thing, but what did Caitlin tell those curious people wondering why there wasn't a father in her picture?

"Well I wouldn't go into it if I didn't know them very well, but I would say a kind man helped my mum have a baby and that's me." If Caitlin's mother Katrina ever responded to the question about where the dad was, she would often say her daughter didn't have a dad.

Caitlin had none of this. She would interject with, "I do have a dad, but he lives in another country." Caitlin continued, "I always felt I have my family but there was a part of me really just wanting to know who he is like deep down inside. Because he's my biological father!" Evidently, there was no way she could let the subject rest. "I've always wanted to know who my biological father is and I've always wanted to know all the siblings. I just wanted to know everybody."

As an open donor, he nominated his details to be released to any donor conceived children once they turned eighteen. He also provided a wealth of information about himself, which was what Katrina and Caitlin used when they began their search for him.

Caitlin said she "always tried to find him because you're only allowed to when you're eighteen. You have to contact the sperm bank and then they will contact the donor. Except I didn't want to wait til I was eighteen so I was just always trying to find him. So recently I have taken DNA tests and my mum has been able to find him".

The day I spoke with Caitlin and Katrina, they had just connected with their donor who was very surprised they were able to track him down. It was a decade sooner than he envisaged but he welcomed the contact. He was also surprised to learn there were a few other children out there. I guess he didn't really believe in his sperm quality or something. I mean, that's what is hopefully going to happen with the sperm you donate to a fertility clinic!

Michael from Adelaide stumbled across his conception story by accident. His mum had been writing memoirs and sending him chapters to proofread. Once on a visit to her home while she was away, he saw some chapters on her computer she'd not yet shared with him. He was curious because they were chapters about him and like most of us, was interested in learning more about himself so began reading. And reading. And then there it was, in black and white on his screen. His whole world as he knew it, cracked wide open. Michael held onto the information for a year before sharing it with his sister, who too was from a donor, albeit a different one to his.

He said "I remember when I found out, thinking it was not something that really happened. Obviously you'd hear about donating sperm and had seen an ad in the paper about being given 25 bucks for your time. It was sort of a concept that Id heard of but certainly not really thought happened, or not to anyone I knew to be conceived in that way. Certainly not myself."

He continued, "my mum had donor sperm through an organised medical system and they encouraged not telling the kids back then, so that was sort of the wisdom. Don't ask. don't tell. In fact she was basically told by the nurse to not even think about it. To put it out of your mind once she had been inseminated. It's kind of best to not think about it. Certainly, not to talk about it or tell your kids. So it was just the culture and it was really not spoken about."

"The other thing is, that back then there weren't really gay people having kids. Well, they were, but it was not talked about and not really accepted in the culture. There weren't gay parents on television and there was no modern family in the 70s. In the 70s, the edgiest show on TV was the 'The Brady Bunch' because the parents were both divorcees. But I think it's just culture, it was a taboo, I suppose, and not being able to have kids was seen as an inadequacy."

"Nowadays, people having trouble conceiving seem to be an increasingly modern day issue that we've become accustomed to, with IVF and people starting to conceive later in life for a lot of reasons. Just infertility seems to be something that we're all very aware of, that in a way 20 or 30 years ago we just didn't talk about it or there was shame about it. Obviously there's no shame and you just do what you do."

I asked Michael what his thoughts were on women having children and prohibiting contact with the donor and siblings. His response:

"It's just selfish! It's thinking about a baby. It's not thinking about a person who is going to become an adult. It's thinking about getting pregnant but that's just the beginning. I think it's just acknowledging that it's thinking beyond the pregnancy and getting pregnant isn't an end game or even an end result and it's not the end of it. It's thinking beyond that and giving your child the respect of a choice of knowing something that is very profoundly part of that child's identity. It's very profound and a big concept. Like where you come from is something that colours your whole sense of who you are. So it's big."

Mr Stork and I discussed early on in my pregnancy how we could create our dibling pride. I had grandiose fantasies of how this could look much like Christian and Juan's modern family blueprint with annual family barbeques and holiday get togethers. Any potential mamas would have to pass both our own requirements. I'd only sign off on them if they were like-minded and aligned with our life values, perspective and also be congruent enough to participate in coffee and play dates from time to time. Maybe we'd even become good friends, be a support system for one another and extend a hand to one another. For him, they'd have to jump through all his rigorous recipient requirement hoops which he initially put me through.

Images of 'Under the Tuscan Sun' came to the forefront of my mind. Specifically, the scene where Diane Lane's character, Frances contemplates the young Polish couple's wedding celebration hosted at her restored villa. Her wish was to one day have a family there and without realising it, her dream came true. It just didn't come in the traditional package that she had limited herself to thinking FAMILY must come in. I get a wave of warm fuzzies every time I visually plonk myself in this movie moment.

However the bigger picture unfolds, for now my little guy and I are our own happy family. His DNA links may extend beyond us, but we are our own complete unit of two.

# Chapter 24

# The Donor Daily

*"Everyone is entitled to his own opinion, but not his own facts."*
*- Daniel P. Moynihan, American politician*

## Down the troll hole – The art of public condemnation

GOSSIP MAGAZINES, BLOGS, SOCIAL PAGES in a newspaper, TV shows and channels of voyeurism aren't something I avoid. I mean, it would be quite a feat for any woman to avoid locking eyes with the people on the cover of magazines while waiting in line at any supermarket checkout aisle.

Having had a minuscule amount of media light shone my way, I found that I was an easy target for the sheer armchair venom waiting on the sidelines to take pot shots. And my choices were under the most extraordinarily vicious microscope.

Occasionally there's been a funny comment or genuinely curious question, but mostly the outpouring of all of the elemental misunderstandings, conflicting beliefs and values, hypocrisy, judgement, untruths and sometimes sheer bloody fear have been attached to my story.

Here is a small sample and a reply if my book hasn't covered it... not something I can do in social media, the press, or a magazine, but here, I can answer knowing that ultimately people will continue to judge, misunderstand and disagree.

Comments are in reference to public interviews I've done or articles I've written that were repurposed by media outlets without factual correction from me. These ones are taken from the Daily Mail and ABC Australian news website, and Facebook pages.

# Selfish Society

*Annie: I am so disappointed in the selfish society we have now. Do any of you ever step back and look at the horrendous big picture you are creating? It is a mess.*

*Annie: That's right - selfish. This is a woman who got to 42 without a commitment to a relationship and now thinks she can commit to a lifelong relationship with a child and is deliberately not thinking of the basic human right of any human to have 2 present parents.*

*Mal: All I can see is another taxpayers burden because this selfish woman is going to be a sole parent. And another non-natural case of a child growing up with no father.*

*Greg: What a waste ....self absorbed person. Sounds like she got to 42 and was desperate. Just hope our tax dollar isn't goin to pay for her motherly dreams. I read some of her blog to see that the efforts she went to, in tryin to get pregnant, including hooking up with her ex. That guy had a lucky escape from child support. While I recognise a need for such generosity in sperm supply as an option for expensive IVF...I feel parenting is more than one person's desire to procreate. Was the promotion/her appearance a marketing stunt on her behalf?*

*Kevin: A very vain person*

Someone also hissed about my baby's impact on population growth.

Jane Goodall has said, "It's our population growth that underlies just about every single one of the problems that we've inflicted on the planet.

If there were just a few of us, then the nasty things we do wouldn't really matter and Mother Nature would take care of it — but there are so many of us."

I lamented it, too, but my one child does not impact the terrible figures; it's large families that do. Jane, along with many other environmental impact experts, is not against people making babies; their message is about

CHAPTER 24 THE DONOR DAILY

promoting smaller families. My one child is a small footprint; we are only half the size of a traditional sized western family.

Professor Cliff can't reiterate enough that our ageing population combined with infertility is going to have massive social and economic ramifications in this country in the next 30 years. We need babies!

## Fatherless Family

*Michael: Can you please weigh up the advantages of a child's life without a father vs the advantages of with a father? Because I can post the real facts, you bunch of ignorant human beings.*

*Henry: No good can come of it. I grew up without a father; there is a void that can't be filled. A feeling my 14 Year old son will never know.*

## General Fear & Hate

*Kelly: What sort of person takes free sperm over the internet?*
*James: A sicko kelly nxt week letz cross breed animals & humans*
*Isis: Someone who is not too fussy.*
*Traude: Desperate one!!!*
*Paradise, Queensland, Australia: Just because you can doesn't mean it's right.*

*Maebe: Ms Hendrix has written a book about her experience and says she also has other projects in the pipeline. Is that the magic pipeline that allows you to be impregnated via social media? I knew you couldn't trust those quiz apps.*

## Name Change

*Barbs: I was with her until she said she changed her name. That's weird.*

## Self Fulfillment

*Wayne: Sometimes buying a dog would solve a lot of problems*

## It's ALL About The Ca-ching $$

*Simon: Should make up a little gift pack with a chocolate and Child support application form....*

*Traude: Simon yes I know! Just wait, I hope all dads have to do it in future....in US they have to...every idiot can make a baby, but why should others financially pay for it...we might have to get a support group together and make it law...*

*Gilly: Baby machines everywhere now eh. Women will never need to get a normal job but live off welfare for life almost as long as they keep having babies eh.lol*

*Opinionated, Brisbane: So does she claim single parent pension?*

## Understanding Fertility & Infertility

*AMK: If you have IUI, you're not medically infertile...*

Again, according to the World Health Organisation (WHO)

"Infertility is a disease of the reproductive system defined by the failure to achieve a clinical pregnancy after 12 months or more of regular unprotected sexual intercourse."

After years of being a relationship with no success followed by three failed IUIs in a row, my fertility clinic considered me medically infertile.

## Potential Donor?

*Graham, Brisbane: I guess a little vial full of tadpoles arrives in the mail? Let me know how you ladies are going. I offer a 7 year warranty with mine. It's also guaranteed colour fast!*

Great. Sign up!

## Playing God

Not surprisingly, some of the biggest critics, sceptics and adversaries of my chosen journey and the similar ones of many other women, are those who align themselves with religions, but in the words of known Christian donor, JLM (John Lyndsay Mayger):

*"I base my actions on my beliefs from God's word....*

*1) Genesis 1: 28 "God said to the man - Be Fruitful! Multiply! Fill the Earth!" all in the vocative. It is hard wired into mankind/womankind to have progeny. No discussion is to be entered into as God directed the first three words to humanity about having children.*

*2) Where a woman's husband dies she is to be impregnated by his brother so that the resulting children will be called the dead man's children. Deut 25:5-10. These children will also care for the widow. Even if the brother was married previously/currently he is to take her as an additional wife, impregnate her NI and care for her children see Book of Ruth and Genesis 38 Judah impregnating his Daughter-in-law with twins. He declares her righteous for NI, adultery (she belonged to Judah's third son) and incest! Many Christians like quoting the Old Testament about killing homosexuals but forget to do the most important things.*

*Jesus emphasised that Christians have a life of "Good Works" and are "chosen before the foundation of the world." I like to think that blood donation: 325 whole blood, Plasma and Platelets, is one of my good works and Masturbation for an IVF clinic in 1978-79 and masturbating from 2003 to now for lesbians et al is another.*

*For me sin is NOT doing bad things, SIN is the failure to do good things. The Anglican Prayer Books says in the Communion Confession "... I have left undone those things which I ought to have done & Done those things which I ought not to have done..."*

> *"A wise man makes his own decisions;*
> *an ignorant man follows the public opinion."*
> *- Grantland Rice, writer*

But for every hundred troll comments, there are a few princely ones. Such as an email from Ian.

A couple of weeks after we were settled back home, I decided to share the arrival of Remy with my Facebook friends. I was surprised to receive this email from Ian the following day. We have a stack of mutual friends and acquaintances, so this news had immediately travelled to him.

*Hi!*

*"Someone told me today, you are extraordinary in every way, you made it happen, you got though the challenges, all healthy I hope.*

*It is simply amazing to me what you have accomplished, and as much as I am not part of your life in any way now, I couldn't imagine a better mum, nor outcome for you.*

*You have a good friends group, you have your family I assume in your corner and more, which is awesome.*

*So much awesomeness for you girl, seriously amazing.."*

*Ian x*

A Message from Mr Stork

*A couple of hours after Remy came into this world, I sent a group text sharing my news and the first photo of him and me with my closest friends. DNA Daddy was included in that list.*

*"It feels amazing to be able to help you achieve your long held dream of finally being a mother. I am so glad you've beaten the loud ticking clock that was ringing in your ears.. Being a parent myself I know what it is like to have a child, the feelings it brings on and the love it brings for the child.*

*Apart from the beautiful emotional feeling of totally gifting a child to you, I pinch myself sometimes that at your age (and mine for that matter) we were able to make it happen and so fast.*

*Maybe the baby gods were just on your side.*

*Congratulations!"*

A message from a member of the public

After I told my story publicly on the ABC's 7.30 news program and the story was printed online, I received a few emails from people who got it. Who got me. This is one that held the same sentiment as the others:

*"Well done Hayley!*

*I have just read your story on abc.net.au and decided to take a couple of minutes to congratulate you for your brave choices to both getting pregnant as a single mother and going public about it.*

*Life does not always go as we would like it to go or plan. You had the courage to take a bold decision and started the path to experience one of the most, if not the most important, life event and status, motherhood. I am a father myself and me and my wife had to go into a lot of trouble to welcome our beautiful daughter. Most people have it easy but we were in our late 30s when we started the long process of achieving parenthood. I am sure you will be a wonderful, devoted and loving mother because the more it takes to reach a goal the more you understand how precious that goal, in this case the ultimate gift of life, is.*

*Secondly I commend the courage you showed to go public with your life experience and encourage/inspire many other women in your situation to follow your choice despite the bigotry or ostracism that some people might have towards the "late" age or the single mother status. There is no age or status that can prevent someone to be a loving and caring parent and any person that would think the opposite, for religious believes or bigotry, does not deserve the time of day. There may be a few haters criticising your choice and actions along the way. If that is going to happen just think at them like some silly and closed-minded people boosting your morale for making you feel much more intelligent and open-minded than them.*

*I am sure you will have lots of love and support from your family and friends and the fact that the donor is an open-minded person like you will help your upcoming bundle of joy to grow up in a loving and caring environment and find his/her own identity in the world.*

*Every effort and hardship will be compensated as soon as you will meet your precious gift, once he/she will smile at you or call you mum for the first time, take his/her first steps and even when crying asking for support when his/her first tooth will come out.*

*This is to tell you that you could not have taken a better decision in your life and people like me are proud of you even if we have not even ever met each other before.*

*Thanks for sharing your inspirational story and good luck for the amazing times ahead of you. You will not regret it one bit.*

*Take care and well done again Hayley!*
*Fabio"*

Oh and a quick update since this book was first published. John Cady is no longer with us and is now only spreading seed across the planet from the sky above (RIP Sir) and SDA Adam is no longer married.

*Chapter 25*

# Looking Back

*"Looking back, of course, that was an insane, irresponsible and stupid choice, but if you don't take your chances then you'll never make your dreams come true and I've no regrets, not one."*
*- Bernard Cornwell, novelist*

*I MAY NOT HAVE KNOWN* what life was like with two parents but I didn't feel I was disadvantaged. I could have blamed my father for not giving us the chance to know him or allowing us to experience being part of a "normal" family but mum ultimately filled both his shoes.

I decided that pushing my child agenda onto a man was not right. I also don't think it's fair no matter how much it hurts, to berate a partner for reading the same book as you but not turning the same page as you at the same time. These fundamental relationship elements need to be thoroughly talked out; a baby needs to go into the life plan. In relationships, it's not so much 'do you want to have a baby' it's got to be 'when do you want to start trying?' Working towards the same family goals are crucial to having them materialise. Otherwise, they can be washed away in a merciless flash flood.

Sure, making these admissions can remain as such—just words. It's the reality of humans and the gift we've been so fortunate to all have the right to not act or change our minds. It sucks. No doubt about it. I'm in constant awe when two people come together who can turn a page at the same pace hitting on all the same text at the same time.

Throughout this wild donor ride, I've been able to go head to head with SHAME. Its poison was rampant throughout my life until the moment my midlife meltdown kicked in. For almost forty years, SHAME has been hitching a ride with me. It was forced upon me second hand through family and societal JUDGEMENT. I never wanted to be seen as less than. Or I can't have something because of where I came from.

I knowingly let SHAME share a spot in the car with all my other voices as I forced my way through life. It sunk many of my SHIPS in order for it to stay alive. It joined forces with FEAR bolstering its presence and solidifying its power. It kept me attached to a story. My tragic childhood story; a story that affected me but wasn't mine to carry the burden of.

Shaking the silence of SHAME, stripping FEAR away, chipping back JUDGEMENT, the three ugly step sisters, for the past few years has been liberating. Comparing myself with set social standards was nothing but torturous. It's hard work upholding the ideals of others when those ideals aren't your own. Nor would I want them to be. Having put myself on this solo parent path, SHAME lost its way. There was no SHAME involved in creating a beautiful little human my way. When I realised SHAME, FEAR and JUDGEMENT would keep him from me, I fell apart. While my food truck adventure was my first step forward in aligning with my message publicly, it took a bunch more years for me to fully pivot. Now I'm no longer afraid to show and share my story with others.

These dark three (shame, fear, judgement) now only existed because they tagged along for the joy ride, hidden or silenced in the backseat. If they were exposed, pushed into the light, they could no longer cause dis-ease or pain. The more I travel down my own rocky road, sharing my story loud and proud, these ugly step sisters are nowhere to be seen.

The thought of going to scans alone may seem lonely to some people. For me, it wasn't at all. I actually didn't consider the notion too much. I focused on what I did have, not what I didn't. And what I did have was a baby in my belly that filled me with such joy.

Also, had I had a man, I would not have shared so much of this with my mother. It has truly been special and memorable. I have given her a gift I could never have imagined would be so fulfilling, a reason for her to wake up at 5am each day! This was such a wonderful gift for both of us.

I'm grateful for how I did this. Truly, this had nothing to do with following my gut, my heart or my mind. It had everything to do with every living cell working together with divine timing knowing I was ready to be a mother. I was born to be one.

As I look back now, I can see how my three most poignant romantic relationships were very telling of who I was at those times in my life. Like growth markers, they served as platforms of which I explored the many facets of myself not only while in them, but before and after each one.

Apart from the very first time I entered a relationship, it seemed I was always just putting myself together again from the last one as I entered a new one. I had been shaped a little differently to share myself with someone. Sometimes I put myself back together better, but sometimes I wasn't quite ready for the bright, shiny new one that was about to enter my little life bubble.

Franz was a silly first love choice but was a really good lifeline at the time. His lifestyle gave me a taste of something bigger and I latched onto that in the best way possible. All the drama that came with my blind fling with Trey represented who and what I dislike most. Self-importance. Selfish wealth. Seen to be scene(y). JUDGEMENT. Worst of all, EGO was in control tooting the bloody horn as I pushed forward on my little media career mission.

Ian landed in my highway lane when EGO had finally abandoned the wheel. I was nearing the end of my thirties and as much as I wanted the big life dream, I also ached for life's simplicities. I think I always did but couldn't yet honour it. My life loves just couldn't fill me up like the pitter patter of tiny feet could. Ian put me on course, not off it. I went there kicking and screaming, but I needed to go through what I did in order to have this baby who I have in my arms today.

I have no regrets. I'm glad I was strong enough to do this and know that I needed to do this to make it true for me. Had I hung on to my relationship with Ian, I wouldn't have Remy. I would be cradling ANGER instead. Holding my miniature miracle in my arms, I am so thrilled I took this path. In some kind of way, I'm glad that it encompassed the gamut of emotions that it did. I truly felt I got to find me in amongst the forest. Had I allowed the three ugly step sisters to steer me off course, I would have been living for others and denying myself what I've always wanted—FAMILY.

*Epilogue*

# Looking Ahead

*"I know not what the future holds, but I know who holds the future."*
*- author unknown*

## My Second Life Act

NEVER, EVER, COULD *I HAVE* imagined waking up at two in the morning to change outfits due to a t-shirt sodden in boob-juice, opposed to being drenched in sweat after some zealous bed action. As I sit on my couch each day, for many hours, both breasts pulsate as one is being head butted, punched, stretched and snapped like an elastic band, then sucked on by the cutest little man I could ever have hoped for. I laugh tears of joy, and sometimes a little pain, as my newborn baby looks up at me with an enormous, gummy smile while my enlarged, throbbing nipple squirts milk in all directions across his face. It's just another priceless moment that I'm racking up being a new mum at 42 years old.

Yesterday's one was even better. Upon rolling into the Mother's Room after having lunch with my wing women Kim and Chez at a shopping mall cafe, I was left gasping for air as I changed his nappy. His ginormous,

202

yellow explosion that made its way right up his back literally had me gagging as I struggled to swiftly extract baby wipes from the packet.

One hand wrangled his feet while I mopped what looked very much like my turmeric latte from the day before. Once I survived that ordeal, I washed my hands and dashed to the car, which I had somehow misplaced. After twenty minutes of zigzagging up and down each lane across two levels, this time losing my own shit, I finally located it. I then loaded us in for the forty minute drive home in peak traffic.

My frustration had me gnawing at my pinky fingernail with the same intensity as a pro boxer hits a heavy punching bag. As I calmed down, I realised something smelled familiar but I couldn't quite place it. Two hands back on the steering wheel, but I still wasn't done with that nail. I gave it another couple of chomps before it dawned on me: that scent was residual turmeric poo-nami. Oh. My. Fucking. God. Suffice it to say, it has been a great nail-biting deterrent ever since.

It already seems a lifetime ago that I was wrestling with the car seat trying to extract it from the car so I could load my newborn into it. It wasn't a one-off fight, however; I couldn't figure out how that damn thing worked for a whole week. The first time I fought with it, was when Mum and I were getting ready for our first car trip outing with bubs. The car seat and I went at it for a whole half an hour. I got all hot and flustered. I even worked up quite a sweat yelling at the bloody thing.

Truth be told, I was swearing like a trooper.

"Sure it's a safety fucking seat," I sneered to myself. "It's safe from me ever fucking using it!"

It took me viewing a YouTube video ten times over the course of the day to figure it out. As I reclaimed my cool, and just before I gave in, all of a sudden something just clicked and the car seat conveniently released from the base.

I've never been more thankful for those kind folks who make these videos for idiots like me. YouTube also came to my rescue when I needed to learn how to pack and unpack the new stroller I had just purchased. I even had to get an impromptu lesson off a young mum in a parking lot who could see how distressed I was when I pulled it out of the boot. I still actually haven't figured out how to do it properly, and I've resigned myself to the fact that I probably won't ever during my kid's early pram phase.

Side note: Until I popped my dear beloved out into this world, I had no idea that there is an all-out 'posh pram posse', but I quickly learned. One day as I was grabbing a coffee at a popular waterside cafe, I noticed a bunch of yummy mummies across from me all rolling with the same trendy brand of stroller. As an 'old mama' who didn't hang with a cool clique, it looked like I had missed the memo on this too. Until that moment, I was pretty chuffed with my bad ass Bugaboo especially since I nabbed it for half price off Gumtree. What a bugger-boo-hoo! My pram was passé and I've been snubbed by patrons of the phooey glam pram clan.

Rewind to several years ago, I was with two of my friends at a high end pop up event for a new lifestyle business on Montana Ave in Santa Monica. I vividly recall an older couple at this opening with their newborn bub in a baby capsule in tow. We could hear them gushing about their new bundle to a couple of women next to us. We avoided an introduction as the three of us were so disinterested in losing our night to a conversation about birth, sleepless nights and breastfeeding.

This was a prime Friday night and we were single. Losing valuable minutes to oohs and aahs would only keep us from potentially meeting 'the one'. Or the 'one right now'. Or even the one to get us to having our very own bundle of joy. The three of us literally stepped over this baby, which was at their feet, barely throwing a glance in their direction as we walked over to the pop-up bar.

Looking back, I can see why those parents were so proud and why that little bundle of joy meant so much to them. The mother glowed; the father stood tall. She was at least ten years older than me, so knowing what I know now, even without knowing their story at all, I can only imagine what they must have gone through to have their baby—reason to bring him out and show him off to the world.

Thank God we didn't engage in conversation with them at the time. That couple would only have thought the things about that earlier version of me that I do today, which makes me cringe.

I couldn't imagine what life would look like without our day being a sing-along. A good chunk of the daylight hours are a constant musical, which picks up where it finished up the night before. EVERYTHING is a song and dance. The song is always out of tune. But it's always on.

Watching my bugalugs throwing his arms and legs about on the living room floor like an upside down turtle, I realise through my baby-making campaign that I succeeded in a couple of things. One, my son.

Two, I have found my purpose. I am now on a mission through the launch of my company Kbuti Group to use human kindness where I can, to be at the centre of all that I do.

Helping others to thrive, starting with and extending to helping those reading this book who need a helping hand for their own path to purpose a new life.

My career, ironically, has finally been covered with a clarity mission and purpose and all because I took these first frightening steps into the unknown.

Having gone through such a long, drawn out break up with Ian, getting my body and mind reproductive, dealing with the fertility clinic failures, searching out a donor online, I couldn't help but share what I'd learned.

Once I found out I was pregnant, I spent the first few months finishing up my book research and then did some rewriting and interviewing for more content until about 7 months in. I told myself that once my cub arrived I'd lose my time and never get it finished, so was extremely focused and motivated. It also helped me stay out of my head.

To be completely honest, I was just trying to remain cautiously optimistic throughout my pregnancy. Until I saw that baby held up by the doctor in the delivery theatre, I did not allow myself to get too attached to the idea that I was really and truly having a baby, and that I was going to be a mother. I was relieved. I could finally breathe again.

Well sort of. Part two of this process had been a success. I am still hoping that a special hu(He)man will sit alongside me at some stage of this journey, but this time with both of us sitting in the backseat of an autonomous car and no one at the wheel.

Well, maybe Remy.

# Glossary

AI: Artificial Insemination
AI+: Artificial Insemination
AF: Aunt Flo/Period
AMA: Advanced Maternal Age (35+)
AMH: Anti-Mullerian Hormone
ART: Assisted Reproductive Treatment
BD: Baby Dance/Intercourse
BFP: Big Fat Positive
BFN: Big Fat Negative
Black Dog: Depression
Bloke: A male species
Boot: Trunk
Box: Vagina
Bugalugs: Baby
Bun Gun: Any sperm-to-uterus transferral device! Needleless
    syringe, penis, soft cup, Stork
Caca: Trouble
CD: Cycle Day
Centrelink: Government Benefits
CM: Cervical Mucus
Cooties: Germs
Conception: the act of creating a person.
CP: Cervical Position
Cryopreservation: Freezing living cells and tissues to preserve
    them
DC: Donor Conceived (person)
DD: Doona Dance/Donor Daddy/DNA Daddy
DD: Dear Daughter
Dibling: Donor Sibling

DMV: Dept of Motor Vehicles

DNA: Deoxyribonucleic Acid

Domance: Donor Romance - The "courting" period.

Donamily: Donor Family

DS: Dear Son

DP: Donor (conceived) Person

DPO: Days Past Ovulation

EDD: Estimated Due Date

Eggies: Ovaries

Embryo: Fertilised Egg

EP: executive Producer in TV

EWCM: Egg White Cervical Mucus

FOMO: Fear Of Missing Out

FSH: Follicle Stimulating Hormone

Geriatric: Old Person

GMO: Genetically Modified Organism

GnRH: Gonadotropin-Releasing Hormone

GP: General Practitioner

Gunga: Weed, Pot, Marijuana

Guppy: Baby

HCG: Human Chorionic Gonadotropin (detected by pregnancy tests)

HI: Home Insemination

HyFosy: Hysterosalpingo-foam sonography

HyCoSy: Hysterosalpingo-contrast-sonography

HPT: Home Pregnancy Test

Hubby: Husband

Hetero: Heterosexual Individual

Hoo-ha: Vagina

HSG: Hysterosalpingogram

Insem: Insemination

IVI: Intra-Vaginall Insemination

ICI: Intra-Cervical Insemination

ICSI: Intracytoplasmic Sperm Injection

IUI: Intrauterine Insemination

IVF: In Vitro Fertilisation

Jiz/Jizz Shiz: Sperm/semen

Juju: Magical or supernatural power

Oocyte: Human Egg

Ovu: Ovulation

LBD: Little Black Dress

LGBTIQ: Lesbian, Gay, Bisexual, Transgender, Intersex and Questioning

LH: Luteinizing/Luteinising Hormone

LMP: Last Menstrual Period

LO: Little One

LP: Luteal Phase

LPD: Luteal Phase Detected

MAMIL: 40+ year old man who cycles regularly

Merch: Merchandise

M/C: Miscarriage

Millennial: People born between 1981 and 1996

Ms. Mew Kus: Cervical Mucus

Nappy: Diaper

NI: Natural Insemination

OBGYN/OB: Gynaecologist

OOP: Out Of Pocket Expenses

OPK: Ovulation Predictor Kit

PI: Partial Insemination

Piss-take: Parody, satire or mockery

POAS: Pee On A Stick

Pram: Stroller

Pronor: Professional Donor

Qld: Queensland, Australia

RE: Reproductive Endocrinologist

Recip: Recipient

SBS Sport: Sport programme broadcast on Special Broadcasting Service (Australia)

SDA: Sperm Donation Australia

Sex Ed: Sex Education

Shaggable: Sexually attractive

Siri: Apple Inc's Virtual Assistant

SO: Significant Other

Soldier: Sperm

Stage Five Clinger: Massive crush on someone
STI: Sexually transmitted Infections (formally diseases)
Swimmers: Sperm
2WW/TWW: Two Week Wait
Taddies: Tadpoles (sperm)
Trackies: Sweat pants
Tracky dacks: Sweat pants
TTC: Trying To Conceive
Tizz - Nervous excitement or agitation
Up The Duff: Pregnant
Vajayjay: Vagina
Viparita Karani: Leg up the wall yoga pose
VO: Voice Overs
WAG: Wives and Girlfriends

# Find Out More

If you want deeper, more succinct advice about how to carve out your own rogue baby making journey, head over to kbuti.com. Here, I share much more comprehensive information to assist you on your path to pregnancy.

Professor Cliff Hawkins
Biohawk
22 Clinker St, Darra QLD 4076
Ph: (+61) 7 3376 9518
E: info@biohawk.com.au
www.biohawk.com.au

Stephen Page
Harrington Family Lawyers
Level 12 – 239 George Street
BRISBANE QLD 4000
Ph: (+61) 7 3221 9544
www.harringtonfamilylawyers.com

Donor Sibling Registry
PH: (+1) 303-258-0902
E: . wendy@donorsiblingregistry.com
www.donorsiblingregistry.com

# Suicide Crisis Support

Australia: Lifeline. Crisis Support and Suicide Prevention - lifeline.org.au - PH: 13 11 14

USA: National Suicide Prevention Lifeline - suicidepreventionlifeline.org - PH: 1-800-273-8255

UK: Samaritans - samaritans.org - PH: 116 123
New Zealand: Lifeline - lifeline.org.nz - PH: 0508 828 865

Canada: Canada Suicide Prevention Service - crisisservicescanada.ca - PH: 1-833-456-4566

South Africa: Lifeline - lifeline.co.za - PH: 0861 322 322

# References

AAP. 2018, Parents reach settlement with IVF clinic after sons were born with genetic condition Fragile X syndrome. The Age. viewed 17 November 2018, http://www.theage.com.au/nsw/parents-sue-ivf-clinic-after-sons-were-born-with-genetic-condition-fragile-x-syndrome-20171113-gzkdil.html.

About Muscular Dystrophy n.d. Muscular Dystrophy Foundation Australia, viewed 17 November 2018, https://mdaustralia.org.au/neuromuscular-condition/about-muscular-dystrophy/.

Aeschylus 1868. The Tragedies of Aeschylos: Life of Aeschylus. Agamemnon. Choephori, or The libation-pourers. Eumenides, London, Strahan & Company.

Alcott, L. M. 2007. An old-fashioned girl, Mineola, N.Y., Dover Publications.

Alshahrani, S., Aldossari, K., Al-Zahrani, J., Gabr, A. H., Henkel, R. & Ahmad, G. 2017. 'Interpretation of semen analysis using WHO 1999 and WHO 2010 reference values: Abnormal becoming normal'. Andrologia, vol. 50, no. 2, pp. e12838.

Australian Bureau of Statistics. 2018, Household Income and Wealth, Australia, 2015-16. Australian Bureau of Statistics. viewed 4 October 2017,http://www.abs.gov.au/ausstats/abs@.nsf/Lookup/by%20Subject/6523.0˜2015-16˜Feature%20Article˜Household%20Debt%20and%20Over-indebtedness%20(Feature%20Article)˜101.

Author Unknown. (I know not what), Attributed to various people including Homer, Greek Philosopher. However, identifying original source could not be established.

Author Unknown, (A bend in the road), Attributed to various people. However, identifying original source could not be established.

Author Unknown: (Not without a shudder), Attributed to various people including Friedrich Schiller. However, identifying original source could not be established. https://en.wikiquote.org/wiki/Talk:Friedrich_Schiller

Australian STI Management Guidelines, 2017, viewed 4 January 2018, http://www.sti.guidelines.org.au

Barry, D. 2016. Best. state. ever. a Florida man defends his homeland, New York, G. P. Putnam's Sons.

Bennett, R. 2016. The Light in the Heart: Inspirational Thoughts for Living Your Best Life, Roy Bennett, quote used with personal permission, Nov 2018.

Bielman, R. 2014. Wild About Her Wingman: A Secret Wishes Novel, Entangled Bliss Books, Entangled Bliss Books, quote used with personal permission, Nov 2018.

Blacketor, P. G. 2009. Riceland, G. Everyday Useful Quotes, Xlibris US.

Buffett, W. Interview, 2017, Warren Buffett - Success is getting what you want, happiness is wanting what you get [Video]. At 31 seconds. https://www.youtube.com/watch?v=m8BOmSLE0RQ: Empower.

Cady, J, 2018. Guide to Natural Insemination. Retrieved from https://naturalinsemination.wordpress.com

Cary Grant 2018. Wikipedia. viewed 10 July 2018, https://en.wikipedia.org/wiki/Cary_Grant.

Cerebral Palsy Alliance. viewed 10 July 2018, https://www.cerebralpalsy.org.au

Chardin, J. 2012. Voyages ... En Perse, Et Autres Lieux de L'Orient. 10 Tom. [And] Atlas... Charleston, SC, Nabu Press.

Cornwell, B, 2018, quote used with permission in personal email from Bernard Cornwell 21 Nov 2018, http://www.bernardcornwell.net

Cystic Fibrosis - What is CF?, viewed 10 July 2018, https://www.cysticfibrosis.org.au/about-cf/what-is-cf

Dalai Lama 2009. The Art of Happiness: A Handbook for Living, New York, NY, Riverhead Books.

DeJoria, John Paul, 2018. Wikipedia. viewed 2 January 2018, https://en.wikipedia.org/wiki/John_Paul_DeJoria.

Department of Human Services 2018, Having a baby. Australian Government. viewed 17 November 2018, https://www.humanservices.gov.au/individuals/subjects/having-baby.

Down Syndrome Australia, What is Down syndrome?, 2018, viewed December 18 2017, https://www.downsyndrome.org.au/what_is_down_syndrome.html#genetic_condition

Dukenfield, W. C. 2016. Fields for President, Taylor Trade Publishing.

Einstein, A. 1955. Old Man's Advice to Youth: 'Never Lose a Holy Curiosity. The Life. I Love a Charade - Sex and The City - Season 5, Episode 8, 2002, HBO, New York, NY. Produced by Darren Star Productions; directed by Michael Engler.

Euripides 1959. Euripides III: Orestes, Iphigenia in Aulis, Electra, The Phoenician women, The Bacchae, New York, NY, Modern Library.

Faulkner, W. 1937. Soldiers' Pay, New York, NY, Sun Dial Press Incorporated.

Fonda, J. 2011, Life's Third Act. TedX Women. viewed February 2018, https://www.ted.com/speakers/jane_fonda_1.

Forbes, B. C. 1922. Forbes epigrams: 1000 Thoughts on Life and Business, New York,, B. C. Forbes publishing company.

Garel, L, 2013, Vogue. Viewed 10 August 2018, https://www.vogue.it/en/uomo-vogue/cover-story/2013/09/cover-louis-garrel

Genetics Home Reference 2018, Sickle cell disease. U.S. Department of Health & Human Services. viewed 17 November 2018, https://ghr.nlm.nih.gov/condition/sickle-cell-disease.

Geraghty, A. A., Lindsay, K. L., Alberdi, G., McAuliffe, F. M. & Gibney, E. R. 2015. 'Nutrition during Pregnancy Impacts Offspring's Epigenetic Status— Evidence from Human and Animal Studies'. Nutrition and Metabolic Insights, vol. 8s1, no., pp. NMI.S29527.

Guppy, 2018, Wikipedia, viewed 8 July 2018, https://en.wikipedia.org/wiki/Guppy.

Haemophilia 2018. Haemophilia Foundation Australia. viewed 17 October 2018, https://www.haemophilia.org.au/about-bleeding-disorders/haemophilia.

Hall, K. 2016, Meet Matt Stone. He's become a dad to up to 100 children in just four years thanks to Facebook. Mama Mia. viewed 9 October 2018, https://www.mamamia.com.au/facebook-sperm-donor/.

Hall, M. 2018, The Saturn Return and Its Significance in Astrology. ThoughtCo. viewed April 2018, https://www.thoughtco.com/what-is-the-return-of-saturn-206368.

Harley, N. 2016, World's most prolific sperm donor - with 800 children - finds clients through Facebook. The Telegraph. viewed 17 November 2018, https://www.telegraph.co.uk/news/health/12097491/Worlds-most-prolific-sperm-donor-with-800-children-finds-clients-through-Facebook.html.

Hart, R., Doherty, D. A., Pennell, C. E., Newnham, I. A. & Newnham, J. P. 2012. 'Periodontal disease: a potential modifiable risk factor limiting conception'.

Human Reproduction, vol. 27, no. 5, pp. 1332-1342. Oh Baby! Names. Viewed 2 January 2018, Above the Fold Interactive, LLC, USA, http://www.ohbabynames.com/meaning/name/hendrix/7466#.W-6jqy9L28U.

Heraclitus, c.540–c.480 bc, Greek philosopher: On the Universe fragment 121 (tr. W. H. S. Jones); see Eliot, Novalis

Herold, D. 2011. Love That Golf: It Can Be Better Than You Think, Whitefish, MT, Literary Licensing, LLC.

Hokey Pokey, 1950, Baker, Laprise, & Macak, Sony/ATV Music Publishing Australia Pty.

Hopper, H. 1952. 'The Times-Picayune, Looking at Hollywood: Jerry Lewis in Golf Yarn by Hedda Hopper'. Chicago Tribune, May 31, p.12.

Howard, C, 2014, NLP Training. Completed Private Course, Ubud, Bali.

Howe, E. W. 1962. The Story of a Country Town, Lanham, MD, Rowman & Littlefield.

Huntington's disease 2018. Huntingtons Queensland. viewed 19 July 2018, https://huntingtonsqld.org.au/huntingtons-disease/what-is-hd/.

Hysterosalpingography, 2018, viewed 28 February 2018, https://en.wikipedia.org/wiki/Hysterosalpingography

Hysterosalpingo-foam sonography, a less painful procedure for tubal patency testing during fertility workup compared with (serial) hysterosalpingography: a randomized controlled trial, 2014, Mijatovic, V., Hompes, P., Out, R., & Dreyer, K, viewed 20 December 2017, https://www.fertstert.org/article/S0015-0282(14)00505-6/fulltext

Is Ed Houben Europe's most virile man? 2014. BBC. viewed 20 August 2018, https://www.bbc.com/news/world-europe-26636166.

James, E. L. 2011. Fifty shades of Grey, New York, Doubleday, a division of Random House, Inc.

Jerry Maguire, 1996, motion picture, Gracie Films. USA. Directed by Cameron Crowe.

Monty Python's The Meaning of Life, 1983, motion picture, Universal Pictures, London, UK. Produced by John Goldstone; directed by Terry Jones. Joyce, J. 2008, Ulysses, Oxford ; New York, Oxford University Press.

Kay, S. 2013, The Type. HuffPost. viewed 9 September 2018, https://www.huffingtonpost.com/sarah-kay/the-type_b_3533002.html.

Kiner, Ralph, used this quip while broadcasting a Mets game, but acknowledged it wasn't original with him. It's a play on the commonplace, "It's not how you win or lose, it's how you play the game"

King, M. L. Jr, 1963, Washington, USA, to conclude his speech at the Lincoln Memorial in the march on Washington.

Layton, J. & Coles, A. 2018, Sperm donor who advertises on Facebook says he's fathered 150 children across America thanks to 'super' seed. Mirror. viewed 17 November 2018, https://www.mirror.co.uk/news/us-news/sperm-donor-who-advertises-facebook-12889072.

Leading Fertility & Reproductive Expertise, IVF Australia, 2018, viewed on November 30 2017, https://www.ivf.com.au

Levine, H., Jørgensen, N., Martino-Andrade, A., Mendiola, J., Weksler-Derri, D., Mindlis, I., Pinotti, R. & Swan, S. H. 2017. 'Temporal trends in sperm count: a systematic review and meta-regression analysis'. Human Reproduction Update, vol. 23, no. 6, pp. 646-659.

Lloyd, J., & Mitchinson, J, 2009,. The QI Book of Advanced Banter (D'Souza, Fr, A.). London: Faber and Faber.

Lownie, A, 2002, John Buchan, Edinburgh, Pimlico. Mamil 2018. Wikipedia. viewed 1 June 2018, https://en.wikipedia.org/wiki/Mamil.

Mann, O. 2018 8/10 - The Inseminator. The Modern Man, Mitch Kennedy interview, viewed 26 August 2018, https://www.modernmann.co.uk/new/inseminator.

Marques-Pinto, A. & Carvalho, D. 2013. 'Human infertility: are endocrine disruptors to blame?'. Endocrine connections, vol. 2, no. 3, pp. R15-R29.

Marriages and Divorces, Australia, 2016 2017, Australian Bureau of Statistics, viewed 6 July 2018, http://www.abs.gov.au/ausstats/abs@.nsf/mf/3310.0.

Marriages in England and Wales: 2014 2017. Office for National Statistics. viewed 6 July 2018, https://www.ons.gov.uk/peoplepopulationandcommunity/birthsdeathsandmarriages/marriagecohabitationandcivilpartnerships/bulletins/marriagesinenglandandwalesprovisional/2014.

Mars, Bruno, 2018, Wikipedia, viewed 10 July 2018, https://en.wikipedia.org/wiki/Bruno_Mars.

Martin, Gerald, 2010. Gabriel García Márquez : a life, New York, Vintage Books.

MGTOW, 2018, viewed 15 April 2018, https://www.mgtow.com

Moynihan, D.P. 1986, in Newsweek 25 August

Mother Teresa of Calcutta 2010. In the Heart of the World: Thoughts, Stories and Prayers, Sydney, ReadHowYouWant.

Non-invasive prenatal testing (NIPT) 2018. Pregnancy, Birth and Baby. viewed 17 November 2018, https://www.pregnancybirthbaby.org.au/non-invasive-prenatal-testing-nipt.

Obama, Barack H, 2018. Wikipedia. viewed 2 January 2018, https://en.wikipedia.org/wiki/Barack_Obama.

Obuchowski, P, 2018, Gutsy Women Win, quote used with permission in personal email from Pat Obuchowski 18 Dec 2018, http://www.GutsyWomenWin.com

Park, A. 2017, Looking on online for sperm donors. ABC Net. viewed 20 November 2017, https://www.abc.net.au/7.30/looking-on-online-for-sperm-donors/9132020.

Patinkin, Mark, 2018, Author, personal declaration on social media, quote used with personal permission Nov 2018, https://www.facebook.com/mark.patinkin.7/

Pseudocyesis: What Exactly Is a False Pregnancy?, American Pregnancy Association, 2018, viewed 10 August 2018, http://americanpregnancy.org/getting-pregnant/pseudocyesis-false-pregnancy/

QFG Handbook, Queensland fertility Group, viewed March 2016

Rodriguez, H, 2018, Cervical Hostility and Regaining Fertility to Get Pregnant, viewed 10 August 2018, http://natural-fertility-info.com/causes-female-infertility.html

Rowling, Joanne K, 2018. Wikipedia. viewed 2 January 2018, https://en.wikipedia.org/wiki/J._K._Rowling.

Salmansohn, K. 2016. Think Happy: Instant Peptalks to Boost Positivity, Berkeley, CA, Ten Speed Press, quote used with personal permission Nov 2018 via email.

Scott, W. 2014. Guy Mannering: For Success, Attitude Is Equally As Important As Ability, A Word To The Wise.

Sexual revolution 2018. Wikipedia. viewed 23 August 2018, https://en.wikipedia.org/wiki/Sexual_revolution.

Sexually Transmitted Diseases (STDs), 2015, viewed October 30 2018, https://www.cdc.gov/std/infertility/

Shedd, J. A. 1928. Salt from My Attic, Portland, ME, The Mosher Press.

Sheetz, K. 2018, Epigenetics For Dummies. Oddyssey Online. viewed 2 January 2018, https://www.theodysseyonline.com/epigenetics-for-dummies.

Tay-Sachs Disease n.d. Brain Foundation. viewed 17 November 2018, http://brainfoundation.org.au/disorders/tay-sachs-disease.

The DSR's 2018 Research Tree Booklet, 2018,. Retrieved from https://www.donorsiblingregistry.com/library/dsr-research

Thoreau, H. D. 1994. Walking, San Francisco, Harper San Francisco.

Unexplained infertility: laparoscopy first or art directly, 2016,American Society For Reproductive Medicine, 106(3), e42, Algergawy, A., Alhalwagy, A., Shehata, A., Salem, H., & Alnaby, A, viewed 10 December 2017, https://www.fertstert.org/article/S0015-0282(16)61545-5/fulltext

United States Divorce Statistics n.d. Bohm Wildish & Matsen, LLP. viewed 17 November 2018, http://www.cadivorce.com/california-divorce-guide/divorce-resources/united-states-divorce-statistics/.

Up in the Air, 2009, motion picture, Paramount Pictures, Hollywood, CA. Produced by Daniel Dubiecki, Jeffrey Clifford, Ivan Reitman & Jason Reitman,; directed by Jason Reitman.

Vandenburg, T. & Braun, V. 2017. "Basically, it's sorcery for your vagina': unpacking Western representations of vaginal steaming'. Culture Health & Sexuality, vol. 19, no. 4, pp. 470-485.

Walsch, Neale Donald 1997, material excerpted from the book Conversations with God, Book 3 ©1997, 2012 By Neale Donald Walsch, quote used with permission from Hampton Roads Publishing c/o Red Wheel/Weiser, LLC Newburyport, MA, redwheelweiser.com.

What is Thalassaemia? n.d. Thalassaemia